Communication Scenarios for the MRCPCH and DCH Clinical Exams

Second Edition

REBECCA CASANS

MBBS, MRCPCH

Specialist Registrar in Paediatrics
James Cook University Hospital
South Tees Hospitals NHS Trust, Middlesbrough

and

MITHILESH LAL

MD, MRCP, FRCPCH

Consultant Paediatrician and Neonatologist
James Cook University Hospital
South Tees Hospitals NHS Trust, Middlesbrough
Royal College Tutor
Examiner, MRCPCH and DCH
Programme Director, Northern Deanery Foundation School

Foreword by

Professor SUNIL K SINHA

MD, PhD, FRCP, FRCPCH

Professor of Paediatrics and Child Health, University of Durham
Consultant Neonatologist, James Cook University Hospital
South Tees Hospitals NHS Trust, Middlesbrough

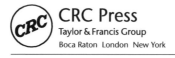

CRC Press
Taylor & Francis Group
Boca Raton London New York

CRC Press is an imprint of the
Taylor & Francis Group, an **informa** business

Radcliffe Publishing Ltd
18 Marcham Road
Abingdon
Oxon OX14 1AA
United Kingdom

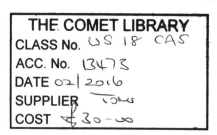
www.radcliffepublishing.com

Electronic catalogue and worldwide online ordering facility.

First Edition 2008

British Library Cataloguing in Publication Data

A catalogue record for this book is available from the British Library.

ISBN-13: 978 184619 494 8

The paper used for the text pages of this book is FSC® certified. FSC (The Forest Stewardship Council®) is an international network to promote responsible management of the world's forests.

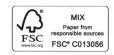

MIX
Paper from
responsible sources
FSC® C013056

Typeset by Pindar NZ, Auckland, New Zealand

Contents

Foreword to second edition

The fact that the second edition of this book is due out within two years of its original publication in itself speaks of the popularity of this book and highlights the importance of the subject. Yet, the desire of the authors for further improvement in this new edition has remained undiminished and they have made several key changes to further enhance its appeal. The highlights of this second edition include a separate chapter on general approach to communication, description of the new DCH clinical examination circuit and the addition of 'new scenarios', making a total of over 100 scenarios, some of which will be particularly relevant to those taking the new DCH examination. No doubt, these changes will appeal to a wider readership and the new edition will continue to play a major role in improving the skills and understanding of effective communication skills.

Sunil K Sinha MD, PhD, FRCP, FRCPCH
Professor of Paediatrics and Neonatal Medicine,
University of Durham & James Cook University Hospital
November 2010

This book is dedicated to my sisters, Claire Lucas and Natalie Dix, my parents, and my husband, Fida Rahman-Casans, for their endless support.
RC

My wonderful daughters, Nikita and Nishita, for their support and encouragement.
ML

Acknowledgement

We would like to thank Professor Sinha for his advice and support during the writing of this book.

List of abbreviations

A&E	Accident and Emergency
AIDS	Acquired immunodeficiency syndrome
ALL	Acute lymphoblastic lymphoma
APLS	Advanced paediatric life support
ASD	Atrial septal defect
BLS	Basic life support
BTS	British Thoracic Society
CF	Cystic fibrosis
CPAP	Continuous positive airway pressure
CT	Computerised tomography
CXR	Chest X-ray
DCH	Diploma in Child Health
DGH	District General Hospital
DKA	Diabetic ketoacidosis
DMSA	Dimercaptosuccinic acid
EBM	Evidence-based medicine
ECG	Electrocardiogram
Echo	Echocardiography
EEG	Electroencephalogram
FY1	Foundation-year 1
GBS	Group B streptococci
GMC	General Medical Council
GP	General practitioner
HIV	Human immunodeficiency virus
HSP	Henoch–Schönlein purpura
IDDM	Insulin-dependent diabetes mellitus
IRT	Immunoreactive trypsin

IV	Intravenous
IVH	Intraventricular haemorrhage
MCUG	Micturating cystourethrogram
MDU	Medical Defence Union
MMR	Measles, mumps, Rubella vaccine
MPS	Medical Protection Society
MRCPCH	Membership of Royal College of Paediatrics and Child Health
MRI	Magnetic resonance imaging
MRSA	Methicillin-resistant *Staphylococcus aureus*
NAI	Non-accidental injury
NEC	Necrotising enterocolitis
NGT	Nasogastric tube
NICE	National Institute for Health and Clinical Excellence
NSAID	Non-steroidal anti-inflammatory drug
OCP	Oral contraceptive pill
PALS	Patient Advice and Liaison Service
PDA	Patent ductus arteriosus
PEG	Percutaneous endoscopic gastrostomy
PICU	Paediatric intensive-care unit
PKU	Phenylketonuria
PS	Pulmonary stenosis
RCPCH	Royal College of Paediatrics and Child Health
RDS	Respiratory distress syndrome
SHO	Senior House Officer
SIDS	Sudden infant death syndrome
SSPE	Sub-acute sclerosing panencephalitis
STI	Sexually transmitted infection
TPN	Total parenteral nutrition
TSH	Thyroid-stimulating hormone
UAC	Umbilical artery catheter
USS	Ultrasound scan
UTI	Urinary tract infection
UVC	Umbilical venous catheter
VSD	Ventricular septal defect
WHO	World Health Organization

Introduction

In its first two years, the first edition of this book has been well-received both in the UK and overseas. Encouraged by this development, this second edition has been updated to include new scenarios (now with a total of over 100 clinical cases) and reflect the recent changes made to the structure of the DCH clinical examination circuit. A separate chapter now focuses upon the general approach to effective communication. This will be useful in any given scenario during day-to-day clinical encounters as well as in the MRCPCH and DCH clinical examinations. We will endeavour to continue to build on what has been achieved so far based on your continuing support and feedback.

Good communication skills are essential for all clinicians, not least paediatricians, who have to deal with the even more challenging aspect of communicating with children, their parents and families. The new MRCPCH clinical examination aims to assess whether candidates have reached the standard of clinical skills expected of a newly appointed specialist registrar. Candidates are expected to demonstrate proficiency in communication, establishing rapport with parents and children, history taking and management planning, physical examination, child development, etc. There are two stations (out of a total of ten) that test the ability to give information to and discuss it with a child, parent (surrogate parent, actor) or a colleague. Success in these two communications skills stations is vital in order to achieve overall success in the clinical examination. It has been our experience through membership clinical teaching as well as examining that prospective candidates are, in general, ill equipped for communication stations. This tends to add to the level of anxiety in most cases. A little help with communication skills will go a long way towards helping candidates to achieve success in the MRCPCH clinical examination.

This book is intended to help candidates who are preparing for the clinical MRCPCH and DCH examinations. It will also be useful to all paediatric trainees in their day-to-day clinical encounters. It is not our intention to provide a textbook of paediatrics or clinical examination. This will no doubt provide a broad framework that can be applied to a whole range of communication scenarios. There are six main patterns of communication scenarios in the membership examination, namely information giving, breaking bad news, consent, critical incidents, ethics and education. We have grouped a range of illustrative examples within each of these six areas. This is by no means an exhaustive list of all possible communication scenarios.

It is not our intention to provide 'model answers.' In fact, one of the greatest challenges of good communication is that it is 'unscripted.' It is not about content delivery, but adapting to a two-way conversation that is tailored to the recipient. The element of unpredictability with regard to specific questions or emotional responses on the part of the recipient makes it challenging. There is no recipe that will work in all situations.

Some examples have specific bullet points relating to key pointers. In others we have merely provided a structure within which to frame your conversation. Candidates are advised to make their own notes in the space provided. This should include notes from your own reading around the topic, particularly any weak areas that you may have identified, to form your own bullet points or structure. Not every scenario included in this book will be encountered in the exam setting. However, if you repeatedly practise this type of communication scenario you will be well equipped to deal with any unfamiliar situations that are presented to you in the clinical examination.

Candidates are advised to go through examples of communication scenarios from the college website (www.rcpch.ac.uk) as well as the mark sheet. They will be marked not just on the process (conduct of interview), but also on the appropriateness of their explanation and the accuracy of the information that they provide. This means that they need to:

▶ select the most appropriate information to communicate
▶ provide information that is correct
▶ explain issues in an appropriate way, without using jargon
▶ respond and adapt to the emotional context of the station.

It is not a test of the amount of information that can be conveyed in 9 minutes. In some scenarios, the task would normally take more than 9 minutes, and may therefore not be completed. Candidates will be penalised for asking irrelevant questions or providing superfluous information.

Finally, candidates should set aside time to team up with like-minded colleagues and get plenty of practice before the exam.

Rebecca Casans
Mithilesh Lal
November 2010

General approach to effective communication: useful tips

The candidate is expected to actively and clearly engage with the patient/parent(s) and colleagues in equal and open dialogue. They should demonstrate the art of *active listening* and be able to communicate verbal and written information in a clear and concise manner.

Indicators of effective communication

Positive indicators	Negative indicators
Checks understanding and summarises effectively	Makes assumptions about understanding
Demonstrates an ability to negotiate effectively	Unable to negotiate effectively
Adapts style of communication to the audience	Does not consider target audience in style of communication
Demonstrates active listening skills	Shows limited evidence of active listening to others
Expresses information clearly and concisely	Has difficulty in expressing information in a way that is easy to understand
Demonstrates empathy, creating a safe and understanding atmosphere	Appears authoritarian and isolated, showing little visible understanding

Breaking bad news
Breaking bad news to either parents/carers or the patient him- or herself is an area that many candidates find challenging. In fact it is something which most clinicians find difficult, as few of them have had much experience in this area.

There are some useful pointers to think about before engaging in any conversation that will involve giving bad news. Candidates may use the *ideas, concerns and expectations* model as a framework for such consultations:[1]

▶ the parent's/patient's **ideas** (baseline understanding of the nature of the problem)
▶ the parent's/patient's **concerns** (specific worries about each problem)
▶ the parent's/patient's **expectations** (what they hope to get out of this consultation, i.e. their agenda).

Preparation and adequate time are essential.
▶ Preparation is the key to a successful discussion.
▶ Always review the clinical details and ensure that you have the correct name for the parents and, even more important, for the child.
▶ Choose the location carefully. It needs to be somewhere where you will not be disturbed, and you should also ensure that you will not be interrupted by bleeper, pager or telephone.
▶ It is important to allow adequate time, as this type of conversation should never be rushed.
▶ Decide who is going to be present, and find out who the parents want to be present at the time of the discussion. Again this requires forward planning.
▶ Set the scene. Explain why you have come to talk to them, and then ask them what they expected to see you about. Do you have the same agenda?
▶ Always assess their understanding first.
▶ Find out how much the parents/child wish to know at this point.
▶ Consider what information the parents wish to discuss in the presence of a young child.
▶ Be aware of the emotions of the parents and/or child throughout the conversation, and acknowledge these as appropriate.
▶ Silence is OK. It can often feel like a long time, but allow natural pauses.
▶ You can stop the conversation at any point and offer the parents/child a break if things get too difficult.
▶ Summarise what you have said and clarify their understanding.
▶ Provide written information and contact details again where appropriate.

▶ Arrange follow-up, particularly to allow the family to ask questions that may have arisen as a result of the discussion.

▶ Importantly, document in the medical notes the details of the conversation and the individuals who were present.

There is no right or wrong way to conduct these conversations. Often listening to colleagues or consultants, particularly those with a special interest in, for example, palliative care or oncology, will give you more confidence in approaching similar cases yourself.

Reference

1 Silverman JD, Kurtz SM, Draper J. *Skills for Communicating with Patients*. Oxford: Radcliffe Medical Press; 1998.

DCH examination flow chart

DCH CLINICAL EXAMINATION CIRCUIT

6 minute Stations   **Cycle One**

X 2

| Communication 1
6 minutes | → | Communication 2
6 minutes | → | Data Interpretation
6 minutes

NEW STATION | → | Structured Oral
6 minutes |

Total time 36 minutes

9 Minute Stations   **Cycle Two**

X 2

| Clinical
Assessment
9 minutes | → | Focused History
& Management
Planning
9 minutes | → | Child
Development
9 minutes | → | Safe Prescribing
9 minutes

NEW STATION |

Total time 48 minutes

RCPCH examination flow chart

MRCPCH CLINICAL CIRCUIT DIAGRAM

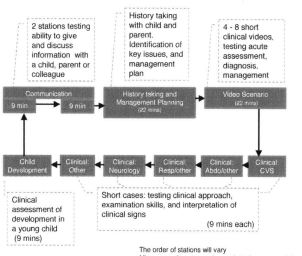

The order of stations will vary
Minor amendments may be made to the proposed circuit.

NB In some overseas centres or smaller exam centres in the UK we may adopt a circuit which spread the circuit across the day and tests the candidates in rotation on the Communication Skills stations, the History taking and Management Planning station and the video station. The Short Clinical and Child Development stations are then tested on in the afternoon.

DCH mark sheet and communication station anchor statement

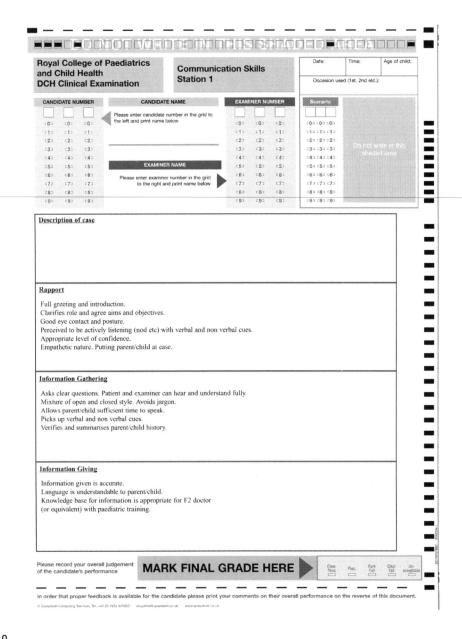

DCH mark sheet and communication station anchor statement (*continued*)

COMMENTS - Communication Skills Station 1

DCH STATION 1 & 2 – COMMUNICATION SKILLS

	Expected standard/CLEAR PASS	PASS	BARE FAIL	FAIL	UNACCEPTABLE
RAPPORT	Full greeting and introduction. Clarifies role and agrees aims and objectives. Good eye contact and posture. Perceived to be actively listening (nod etc) with verbal and non-verbal. Appropriate level of confidence. Empathetic nature. Putting parent/child at ease.	Adequately performed but not fully fluent in conducting interview	Incomplete or hesitant greeting and introduction. Inadequate identification of role, aims and objectives. Poor eye contact and posture. Not perceived to be actively listening (nod etc) with verbal and non-verbal cues. Does not show appropriate level of confidence, empathetic nature or putting parent/child at ease.	Significant components omitted or not achieved	Dismissive of parent/child concerns. Fails to put parent or child at ease.
INFORMATION GATHERING	Asks clear questions. Patient & examiner can hear & understand fully. Mixture of open & closed style. Avoids jargon. Allows parent/child sufficient time to speak. Picks up verbal & non-verbal cues. Verifies & summarises parent/child history.	Questions reasonable and cover all essential issues but may omit occasional relevant but less important points. Overall approach structured. Appropriate style of questioning responsive to parent/child. Summarises history.	Misses relevant information which if known would make a difference to the management of the problem. Excessive use of closed instead of open questions. Uses medical jargon occasionally. Misses verbal or non-verbal cues. Summary inaccurate / incomplete.	Asks closed questions instead of open questions. Questions poorly comprehended by parent/child. Inappropriate use of medical jargon. Inappropriately interrupts parent/child. Hasty approach. Does not seek views of parent or child. Poorly structured interview.	Shows no regard for parent or child's feelings. No verification or summarising.

The final mark for each station is based upon the expert assessment of each candidate's performance, clinical ability and knowledge. These Anchor statements provide a list of the components which contribute to judging a candidates performance. The importance or relevance of the individual component will vary from station to station

RCPCH mark sheet and communication station anchor statements

Royal College of Paediatrics and Child Health		Communication 1	Date:	Time:	Age of child:
MRCPCH Clinical Examination			Occasion used (1st, 2nd etc.):		

CANDIDATE NUMBER	CANDIDATE NAME	EXAMINER NUMBER	Scenario No.

Please enter candidate number in the grid to the left and print name below

c0ɔ c0ɔ c0ɔ
c1ɔ c1ɔ c1ɔ
c2ɔ c2ɔ c2ɔ
c3ɔ c3ɔ c3ɔ
c4ɔ c4ɔ c4ɔ
c5ɔ c5ɔ c5ɔ
c6ɔ c6ɔ c6ɔ
c7ɔ c7ɔ c7ɔ
c8ɔ c8ɔ c8ɔ
c9ɔ c9ɔ c9ɔ

EXAMINER NAME

Please enter examiner number in the grid to the right and print name below

Degree of co-operation of child

Compliant

Hesitant

Unwilling

FOR FEEDBACK PURPOSES MARK THE PERFORMANCE IN EACH SECTION: **Station 1**

Description of scenario

Conduct of Interview   Please mark here ———→   Clear Pass | Pass | Bare Fail | Clear Fail | Un-acceptable

Introduction, clarifies role
Agrees aims and objective
Rapport
Empathy and respect

Appropriate explanation and negotiation   Please mark here ———→   Clear Pass | Pass | Bare Fail | Clear Fail | Un-acceptable

Clear explanation, no jargon
Assesses prior knowledge of patient
Appropriate questioning style
Explores and responds to concerns and feelings
Summarises and checks understanding

Accuracy of information given   Please mark here ———→   Clear Pass | Pass | Bare Fail | Clear Fail | Un-acceptable

Appropriate selection of information
Accuracy of information

Please record your overall judgement of the candidate's performance   **MARK FINAL GRADE HERE** ▶   Clear Pass | Pass | Bare Fail | Clear Fail | Un-acceptable

In order that proper feedback is available for the candidate please print your comments on their overall performance on the reverse of this document.

© Speedwell Computing Services, Tel: +44 (0) 1621 840840   enquiries@speedwell.co.uk   www.speedwell.co.uk

STANDARDS FOR ASSESSMENT: COMMUNICATION STATION

Conduct of Assessment	A candidate will demonstrate:
	an understanding of the roles and responsibilities of paediatricians
	effective responses to challenge, complexity and stress in paediatrics
	effective skills in three-way consultation and examination
	an understanding of equality and diversity in paediatric practice
	ethical personal and professional practice

Appropriate explanation and negotiation	
	an understanding of effective communication and interpersonal skills with children of all ages
	empathy and sensitivity and skills in engaging the trust of and consent from children and their families
	an understanding of listening skills
	Or effective communication and interpersonal skills with colleagues (if communication with colleague not patient or family)
	Or professional respect for the contribution of colleagues in a range of roles in paediatric practice (if communication with colleague not patient or family)

Accuracy of information given	
	knowledge of the science- base for paediatrics (as outlined in the *Framework of Competences for Level 1 in Paediatrics*)
	knowledge of common and serious paediatric conditions and their management
	an understanding of basic skills in giving information and advice to young people and their families

Please turn over for more detailed advice on how to interpret if a candidate has reached these standards

The final mark for each station is based upon the expert assessment of each candidate's performance, clinical ability and knowledge. These Anchor statements provide a list of the components which contribute to judging a candidates performance. The importance or relevance of the individual component will vary from station to station.

ANCHOR STATEMENTS: COMMUNICATION

	Expected standard / CLEAR PASS	PASS	BARE FAIL	CLEAR FAIL	UNACCEPTABLE
Conduct of interview	Full greeting and introduction. Clarifies role and agrees aims and objectives. Good eye contact and body language. Perceived to be actively listening (nod etc) with verbal and non-verbal. Patient and examiner can hear and understand fully. Appropriate level of confidence. Empathetic nature and shows respect. Allows parent/patient sufficient time to speak. Responds appropriately to concerns and emotional needs. Picks up verbal and non-verbal cues.	Overall approach structured. Appropriate style of interview responsive to parent/patient. Verbal and non-verbal skills are at an acceptable level. Minor problems with confidence or delivery of message.	Inadequate identification of role, aims and objectives. Excessive use of closed questions. Fails to respond appropriately to parent/patient concerns. Poor eye contact and body language. Not perceived to be actively listening (nod etc) with verbal and non-verbal cues.	Fails to identify or respond to parent/patient concerns. Unsatisfactory in several components.	Ignores or is dismissive of parent/patient concerns. Lack of civility or politeness. Rudeness or arrogance. Inappropriate manner including flippancy.
Appropriate explanation and negotiation	Clear explanation avoiding jargon. Explores subject's prior knowledge, ideas, concerns, expectations and feelings. Assesses prior knowledge. Asks clear questions with appropriate use of open and closed style. Summarises, checks understanding and concludes the interview appropriately.	Misses minor cues. Generally jargon free. Adequate exploration of subject's knowledge and views. Summary with important details.	Uses medical jargon without explanation. Poor summary. Misses important points or makes too many minor errors.	Communication ineffective in transferring the important information. Poor response to cues. No summary or summary contains significant inaccuracies or is wrong.	**Behavioural:** Arrogant lack of negotiation skills. **Medical Knowledge / Competence:** Serious or dangerous deficiencies in facts explained or method of explanation.
Accuracy of information given	Conveys appropriately selected and accurate information. Information is correct in all-important detail. It is explained in a way that is likely to be understood, and steps are taken to ensure that the important messages have been understood.	Interview covers all essential issues but may omit occasional relevant but less important points.	Major important inaccuracies or too many minor inaccuracies in information given. Poor attempt to ensure understanding.	Significant components omitted or not achieved. Important or numerous inaccuracies in information given.	**Behavioural:** Potentially dangerous information given. **Medical Knowledge / Competence:** Serious inaccuracies in information given.

The final mark for each station is based upon the expert assessment of each candidate's performance, clinical ability and knowledge. These Anchor statements provide a list of the components which contribute to judging a candidates performance. The importance or relevance of the individual component will vary from station to station.

DCH examination examples

DCH COMMUNICATION SKILLS SCENARIO

This station assesses your ability to give information to a parent/patient.

*This is a 6-minute station. You will have 3 minutes beforehand to read this sheet and prepare yourself. You may take the sheet with you into the station, **but you must return it at the end.***

Role: A GP working in a small rural market town.

You will be talking to: Jane Smith, the teenage single mother of 18-month-old Jason.

Setting: GP surgery.

Task: To explore her concerns about febrile convulsions.

YOU ARE NOT EXPECTED TO GATHER THE REST OF THE MEDICAL HISTORY DURING THIS CONSULTATION.

DCH COMMUNICATION SKILLS SCENARIO

ROLE PLAYER INFORMATION

*This is a 6-minute station consisting of spoken interaction between you and the candidate. You will have 3 minutes beforehand to read this sheet and prepare yourself. You may take the sheet with you into the station, **but you must return it at the end**.*

Role: Jane Smith, aged 18 years, the mother of Jason, aged 18 months, who was recently admitted to the local district general hospital following a convulsion. You were told that this was a 'febrile convulsion' and that it was caused by Jason's high fever with a respiratory infection. You have been told to watch out for future sudden high temperatures, and have been reassured that this is unlikely to happen again. You have been given advice about measures to control high temperature.

Your general feelings:
- You are terrified that this may happen again, as you thought Jason was going to die.
- You have lost all confidence as a young single parent, and are concerned about the new out-of-hours arrangements for requesting emergency help.
- You are still worried that your child may be epileptic.

After the doctor has explained the situation to you, your feelings and further questions are:
- What is a febrile convulsion?
- How do you know that my child is not epileptic?
- What are the risks of this occurring again?
- What should I do if he has a high temperature?
- Does he need drugs to prevent this from occurring?
- Has he been brain damaged?

DCH COMMUNICATION SKILLS SCENARIO

The examiner should be given both the candidate sheet and the role player sheet.

This is a 6-minute station consisting of spoken interaction between the candidate and the role player. You should remain silent during the examination time.
If the candidate finishes early, you should check that they have finished. If this is the case, they should remain in the room until the session has ended.

GUIDE NOTES TOWARDS EXPECTED STANDARD

Examiner marking criteria:

The candidate should be able to:

- clearly explain febrile convulsions
- show that there is a good long-term prognosis
- show that there is no link with epilepsy
- show empathy for parent concerns
- explain preventative management.

RCPCH examination examples
RCPCH Example 1

MRCPCH COMMUNICATION SKILLS SCENARIO

CANDIDATE INFORMATION

This station assesses your ability to obtain consent for a medical procedure.

This is a 9-minute station consisting of spoken interaction. You will have up to 2 minutes before the start of the station to read this sheet and prepare yourself. You may make notes on the paper provided.

When the bell sounds you will be invited into the examination room. Please take this instruction sheet with you. The examiner will not ask questions during the 9 minutes but will warn you when you have approximately 2 minutes left.

You are not required to examine a patient.

The encounter should be focussed on the task; you will be penalised for asking irrelevant questions or providing superfluous information. You will be marked on your ability to communicate, not the speed with which you convey information. You may not have time to complete the communication.

Role: An SpR working in a paediatric ward.

You will be talking to: Helen Jones, the mother of Tony, a 5 year-old boy with signs of suspected meningitis.

Background Information: He has been miserable for a few days, is off-colour, feverish and has a headache. You decide that he needs a lumbar puncture.

Task: To seek verbal consent for this procedure.

YOU ARE NOT EXPECTED TO GATHER THE REST OF THE MEDICAL HISTORY DURING THIS CONSULTATION

19

MRCPCH COMMUNICATION SKILLS SCENARIO

ROLE PLAYER INFORMATION

This is a 9-minute station consisting of spoken interaction between you and the candidate. There is no discussion with the examiner.

You are: Helen Jones, the parent of Tony, a 5 year-old boy.

Background Information: Tony has been miserable for a few days. He is off-colour, feverish and has a headache. You have never seen him quite so unwell.

Tony is the eldest of 3 children.

Your general feelings:

- Anxiety about Tony's illness.
- You don't want him subjected to more painful tests and distress.

After the doctor has explained the situation to you, your further questions might include:
- What does it involve?
- Would it hurt, and could he have an anaesthetic?
- What can be done to reduce the pain?
- Is it dangerous, what side effects are there?
- When will I know the result?
- What if he doesn't have it done, can't you treat him anyway?

The main thing is to be CONSISTENT with your story and emotional response with each candidate.

MRCPCH COMMUNICATION SKILLS SCENARIO

This station assesses the candidate's ability to obtain consent for a medical procedure.

This is a 9-minute station consisting of spoken interaction between the candidate and the role-player. You should remind the candidate when 2 minutes remain otherwise you should remain silent during the examination time.

If the candidate finishes early, you should check that they have finished. If yes, they should remain in the room until the session has ended.

INFORMATION GIVEN TO CANDIDATE:

Role: An SpR working in a paediatric ward.

You will be talking to: Helen Jones, the mother of Tony, a 5 year-old boy with signs of suspected meningitis.

Background Information: He has been miserable for a few days, is off-colour. feverish and has a headache. You decide that he needs a lumbar puncture.

Task: To seek verbal consent for this procedure.

INFORMATION GIVEN TO ROLE PLAYER:

You are: Helen Jones, the parent of Tony, a 5 year-old boy.

Background Information: Tony has been miserable for a few days. He is off-colour, feverish and has a headache. You have never seen him quite so unwell.

Tony is the eldest of 3 children.

Your general feelings:

- Anxiety about Tony's illness.
- You don't want him subjected to more painful tests and distress.

GUIDANCE TOWARDS EXPECTED STANDARD:

- Reassurance of parent.
- Clear explanation about LP - why is it necessary and what is involved.
- Explain about analgesia.
- Explain what to expect afterwards.
- Explain risks – infection, leak, headache, technically unsuccessful.
- Explain benefits – confirm diagnosis and management. selection of treatment, length of treatment, follow-up arrangements.

MRCPCH COMMUNICATION SKILLS SCENARIO

Please use this sheet to make a list of the criteria you have used in this station to decide if a candidate is a clear pass, pass, bare fail or clear fail and hand it to the host examiner when you have completed the circuit.

CLEAR PASS

PASS

BARE FAIL

CLEAR FAIL

RCPCH Example 2

MRCPCH COMMUNICATION SKILLS SCENARIOS

CANDIDATE INFORMATION

This station assesses your ability to deal with a clinical problem.

This is a 9-minute station consisting of spoken interaction. You will have up to 2 minutes before the start of the station to read this sheet and prepare yourself. You may make notes on the paper provided.

When the bell sounds you will be invited into the examination room. Please take this instruction sheet with you. The examiner will not ask questions during the 9 minutes but will warn you when you have approximately 2 minutes left.

You are not required to examine a patient.

The encounter should be focussed on the task; you will be penalised for asking irrelevant questions or providing superfluous information. You will be marked on your ability to communicate, not the speed with which you convey information. You may not have time to complete the communication.

You are: An SpR in paediatrics.

Setting: Side room of paediatric ward during a Sunday morning ward round.

You will be talking to: Sally Jones, the mother of David Jones, a 5 week-old baby who was born at term, birth weight 3.5 kg. You have not previously been involved in this baby's care.

Background: David is being investigated for prolonged conjugated jaundice. During the night David has become drowsy and is not feeding and has been having brief periods of apnoea and is requiring supplemental oxygen to maintain his saturations at more than 90%.

You have noted that David was meant to have been prescribed Phenobarbital (phenobarbitone) 15 mg once a day, two days previously but instead has been given 75mg once daily as the writing on the prescription was misinterpreted.

His jaundice started on the second day of life. He was given phototherapy treatment in hospital for days 2-5 but has been jaundiced ever since. He was initially breast fed but his mother's milk dried up.

Task: To talk to Mrs. Jones about the prescribing error and its effects on her son.

YOU ARE NOT EXPECTED TO GATHER THE REST OF THE MEDICAL HISTORY DURING THIS CONSULTATION

MRCPCH COMMUNICATION SKILLS STATION

ROLE PLAYER INFORMATION

This is a 9-minute station, consisting of spoken interaction between you and the candidate. There is no discussion with the examiner.

You are: Sally Jones, the mother of David Jones a 5 week-old baby being investigated for prolonged jaundice. This started on the second day of life. He was given phototherapy (fluorescent light) treatment in hospital for days 2-5 but has been jaundiced ever since. You took him home one week after birth.

You breast-fed him for two weeks but your milk dried up.

He has been started on a drug as part of his investigations but unfortunately has been given 5 times the intended dose.

David is your first child. His current admission to hospital has been for 2 days. You have noticed that he is very sleepy.

David has not eaten today. He is jaundiced and has stopped breathing briefly. He is currently receiving oxygen via a tube under his nose and is on a saturation monitor.

Your general feelings:
- You show controlled anger.
- You want to know why this has happened.

After the doctor has explained the situation to you, your feelings and further questions are:
- Why is he now on oxygen?
- What are the potential problems/side effects?
- Will it delay the investigations for his jaundice?
- What will be done by the hospital to prevent it happening again?

What to expect from the candidate, and how to respond:
- Offered an apology.
- An explanation of the hospital's complaints procedure

The main thing is to be CONSISTENT with your story and emotional response with each candidate.

MRCPCH COMMUNICATION SKILLS STATION

EXAMINER INFORMATION (page one)

This station assesses the candidate's ability to deal with a clinical problem.

This is a 9-minute station consisting of spoken interaction between the candidate and the role-player. You should remind the candidate when 2 minutes remain otherwise you should remain silent during the examination time.

If the candidate finishes early, you should check that they have finished. If yes, they should remain in the room until the session has ended.

INFORMATION GIVEN TO CANDIDATE:

You are: An SpR in paediatrics.

Setting: Side room of paediatric ward during a Sunday morning ward round.

You will be talking to: Sally Jones, the mother of David Jones, a 5 week-old baby who was born at term, birth weight 3.5 kg. You have not previously been involved in this baby's care.

Background: David is being investigated for prolonged conjugated jaundice. During the night David has become drowsy and is not feeding and has been having brief periods of apnoea and is requiring supplemental oxygen to maintain his saturations at more than 90%.

You have noted that David was meant to have been prescribed Phenobarbital (phenobarbitone) 15 mg once a day, two days previously but instead has been given 75mg once daily as the writing on the prescription was misinterpreted.

His jaundice started on the second day of life. He was given phototherapy treatment in hospital for days 2-5 but has been jaundiced ever since. He was initially breast fed but his mother's milk dried up.

Task: To talk to Mrs. Jones about the prescribing error and its effects on her son.

INFORMATION GIVEN TO ROLE PLAYER:

You are: Sally Jones, the mother of David Jones a 5 week-old baby being investigated for prolonged jaundice. This started on the second day of life. He was given phototherapy (fluorescent lights) treatment in hospital for days 2-5 but has been jaundiced ever since. You took him home one week after birth.

You breast-fed him for two weeks but your milk dried up.

He has been started on a drug as part of his investigations but unfortunately has been given 5 times the intended dose.

David is your first child. His current admission to hospital has been for 2 days. You have noticed that he is very sleepy.

MRCPCH COMMUNICATION SKILLS STATION

EXAMINER INFORMATION (page one)

This station assesses the candidate's ability to deal with a clinical problem.

This is a 9-minute station consisting of spoken interaction between the candidate and the role-player. You should remind the candidate when 2 minutes remain otherwise you should remain silent during the examination time.

If the candidate finishes early, you should check that they have finished. If yes, they should remain in the room until the session has ended.

David has not eaten today. He is jaundiced and has stopped breathing briefly. He is currently receiving oxygen via a tube under his nose and is on a saturation monitor.

Your general feelings:
- You show controlled anger.
- You want to know why this has happened.

GUIDE NOTES TOWARDS EXPECTED STANDARD:

- Appropriate conduct of interview.
- An explanation to the parents of how the error occurred.
- To apologise for the reported mistake.
- To recap the situation and to invite parents' questions about the possible toxic effects to David and how these will be monitored.
- To detail the actions necessary which will include:
  o notification of an adverse incident to the Hospital Trust.
  o to document fully in the medical records of the patient the prescribing error and actions taken.
- Closure – reassurance, final apology.

MRCPCH COMMUNICATION SKILLS SCENARIO

Please use this sheet to make a list of the criteria you have used in this station to decide if a candidate is a clear pass, pass, bare fail or clear fail and hand it to the host examiner when you have completed the circuit.

CLEAR PASS

PASS

BARE FAIL

CLEAR FAIL

RCPCH Example 3

MRCPCH COMMUNICATION SKILLS STATION

CANDIDATE INFORMATION

This station assesses your ability to address a father about his worries regarding his son's illness.

This is a 9-minute station consisting of spoken interaction. You will have up to 2 minutes before the start of the station to read this sheet and prepare yourself. You may make notes on the paper provided.

When the bell sounds you will be invited into the examination room. Please take this instruction sheet with you. The examiner will not ask questions during the 9 minutes but will warn you when you have approximately 2 minutes left.

You are not required to examine a patient.

The encounter should be focussed on the task; you will be penalised for asking irrelevant questions or providing superfluous information. You will be marked on your ability to communicate, not the speed with which you convey information. You may not have time to complete the communication.

Role: An SpR.

Setting: Outpatient department of your hospital.

You are talking to: The father of a 10.5 year-old boy who is a known case of Down syndrome.

Background information: Abdulla is a 10.5 year-old boy with Down's syndrome (chromosome trisomy 21 – nondysjunction). He was diagnosed at the age of 3 months to have an AV canal defect. Banding was done at age of 3 months and then total correction was carried out at the age of 1.5 years. At the age of 3 years, he was referred to the Endocrine Unit because of discovery of autoimmune hypothyroidism and is on treatment.

Any other information: He is growing at the 3rd centile in height while his weight is at the 50th centile. At the age of 4 years, he developed extensive frontal and temporal alopecia for which he received treatment from the dermatologist with some improvement. He has mild mental retardation but is not in education since his father does not think that he is capable of being in a regular school.

Task: Identify father's current concerns about the patient's clinical condition and future plans and prognosis.

YOU ARE NOT EXPECTED TO GATHER THE REST OF THE MEDICAL HISTORY

MRCPCH COMMUNICATION SKILLS STATION

ROLE PLAYER INFORMATION

This is a 9-minute station consisting of spoken interaction between you and the candidate. There is no discussion with the examiner.

You are: The father of 3 children with the eldest being Abdulla (aged 10.5 years) who was diagnosed to have Down's syndrome at birth.

Background information: Chromosomal analysis done for you and your wife was found to be normal. Your younger children are normal.

Abdulla had heart failure due to a congenital heart defect (AV canal defect) and banding at the age of 3 months and then total correction was done at the age of 1.5 years. He is currently not on treatment for the heart.

At the age of 3 years, Abdulla's thyroid functions were checked during a visit to the Developmental Department and he was found to have hypothyroidism. He was referred to the Endocrine Unit and was started on thyroid replacement therapy to which he is compliant. Abdulla has a small penis but both testes are in the scrotum.

At the age of 4 years, Abdulla developed extensive hair loss at the front and side of the scalp. He received treatment from the dermatologist with some improvement.

Your son is not at school because you had thought that his mild mental retardation would not allow him to be in a regular school. Now you are reconsidering education prospects for Abdulla.

Your general feelings:
* You are unsure and worried about the future of your child.

After the doctor has explained the situation to you, your feelings and possible further questions may be:

* Risk of recurrence for future children?
* Schooling prospects for Abdulla.
* Cause of your son's hair loss and if it will ever grow again.
* Any special precaution regarding Abdulla's cardiac status?
* You want to know if your son can get married and have children.

The main thing is to be CONSISTENT with your story and emotional response with each candidate.

MRCPCH COMMUNICATION SKILLS SCENARIO

EXAMINER INFORMATION (page one)

This station assesses the candidate's ability to address a father about his worries regarding his son's illness.

This is a 9-minute station consisting of spoken interaction between the candidate and the role-player. You should remind the candidate when 2 minutes remain otherwise you should remain silent during the examination time.

If the candidate finishes early, you should check that they have finished. If yes, they should remain in the room until the session has ended.

INFORMATION GIVEN TO CANDIDATE:

Role: An SpR.

Setting: Outpatient department of your hospital.

You are talking to: The father of a 10.5 year-old boy who is a known case of Down syndrome.

Background information: Abdulla is a 10.5 year-old boy with Down's syndrome (chromosome trisomy 21 – nondysjunction). He was diagnosed at the age of 3 months to have an AV canal defect. Banding was done at age of 3 months and then total correction was carried out at the age of 1.5 years. At the age of 3 years, he was referred to the Endocrine Unit because of discovery of autoimmune hypothyroidism and is on treatment.

Any other information: He is growing at the 3rd centile in height while his weight is at the 50th centile. At the age of 4 years, he developed extensive frontal and temporal alopecia for which he received treatment from the dermatologist with some improvement. He has mild mental retardation but is not in education since his father does not think that he is capable of being in a regular school.

Task: Identify father's current concerns about the patient's clinical condition and future plans and prognosis.

INFORMATION GIVEN TO ROLE PLAYER:

You are: The father of 3 children with the eldest being Abdulla (aged 10.5 years) who was diagnosed to have Down's syndrome at birth.

Background information: Chromosomal analysis done for you and your wife was found to be normal. Your younger children are normal.

Abdulla had heart failure due to a congenital heart defect (AV canal defect) and banding at the age of 3 months and then total correction was done at the age of 1.5 years. He is currently not on treatment for the heart.

At the age of 3 years, Abdulla's thyroid functions were checked during a visit to the Developmental Department and he was found to have hypothyroidism. He was referred to the Endocrine Unit and was started on thyroid replacement therapy to which he is compliant. Abdulla has a small penis but both testes are in the scrotum.

MRCPCH COMMUNICATION SKILLS SCENARIO

This station assesses the candidate's ability to address a father about his worries regarding his son's illness.

This is a 9-minute station consisting of spoken interaction between the candidate and the role-player. You should remind the candidate when 2 minutes remain otherwise you should remain silent during the examination time.

If the candidate finishes early, you should check that they have finished. If yes, they should remain in the room until the session has ended.

At the age of 4 years, Abdulla developed extensive hair loss at the front and side of the scalp. He received treatment from the dermatologist with some improvement.

Your son is not at school because you had thought that his mild mental retardation would not allow him to be in a regular school. Now you are reconsidering education prospects for Abdulla.

Your general feelings:
- You are unsure and worried about the future of your child.

GUIDE NOTES TOWARDS EXPECTED STANDARD

Examiner marking criteria:
- Whether the candidate can sympathetically but firmly engage with the father.
- Ability to explain
  - The risks of recurrence in Trisomy 21.
  - That the child should go to school for improving his developmental and mental capabilities. Special schools are available for children of special needs and developmental challenges.
  - The possibility to link alopecia areata as an autoimmune disease to Hashimoto thyroiditis
- The ability to realize the need for sub acute bacterial endocarditis prior to dental procedures.
- The ability to realize that Down Syndrome males are infertile

MRCPCH COMMUNICATION SKILLS SCENARIO

Please use this sheet to make a list of the criteria you have used in this station to decide if a candidate is a clear pass, pass, bare fail or clear fail and hand it to the host examiner when you have completed the circuit.

CLEAR PASS

PASS

BARE FAIL

CLEAR FAIL

1: Information giving

(e.g. please tell this mother about the diagnosis)

....

This is a 9-minute station consisting of spoken interaction. You will have up to 2 minutes before the start of the station to read this sheet and prepare yourself. You may make notes on the paper provided.

When the bell sounds you will be invited into the examination room. Please take this instruction sheet with you. The examiner will not ask questions during the 9 minutes, but will warn you when you have approximately 2 minutes left.

You are not required to examine a patient.

The encounter should be focused on the task: you will be penalised for asking irrelevant questions or providing superfluous information. You will be marked on your ability to communicate, not the speed with which you convey information. You may not have time to complete the communication.

....

Role: Paediatric registrar.

Setting: Outpatient clinic in a busy DGH.

You are talking to: Mr and Mrs Hope, parents of 3-year-old Lillie.

Background information: Lillie is a 3-year-old girl who was recently admitted to the ward with a new diagnosis of insulin-dependent diabetes. She initially required insulin and fluids intravenously, but has now been discharged home on subcutaneous insulin four times a day. Her parents are managing very well and have met the diabetes team, including the consultant, the dietitian and the children's specialist diabetic nurse. As part of the education package that has been developed for newly diagnosed diabetics, Lillie's parents will be attending clinic today to learn about the pathophysiology of diabetes. This is to aid their understanding of their daughter's condition.

Task: Please discuss the pathophysiology of insulin-dependent diabetes with Lillie's parents.

Points to consider:

▶ Ask how Lillie is doing.
▶ Ask how they are doing as a family. Acknowledge that it must have been a shock for them all and that it is a difficult diagnosis to understand.
▶ Set the scene for today's meeting. You want to try to explain some of the theory behind diabetes, which will hopefully help the parents to understand Lillie's condition more easily.
▶ Invite them to ask questions at any time.
▶ There is a lot of information that you could give them now. Practise this so that you have an explanation which you can easily provide for non-medics.
▶ Start off by explaining the physiology of *glucose homeostasis* (i.e. blood glucose levels are tightly controlled by a balance between food intake and insulin release).
▶ The commonest cause of diabetes in childhood is type 1 autoimmune diabetes. Give a basic explanation of the term '*autoimmune.*'
▶ The annual incidence of the condition is 20 per 100 000 children, and it is increasing.
▶ Diabetes is a metabolic disorder due to a disturbance in insulin function.
▶ Explain the actions of *insulin.*
▶ Autoimmune destruction of the beta-cells of the pancreas leads to a deficiency in insulin secretion. Break this information down and explain it, using diagrams to help.
▶ The clinical effects of low insulin levels, including effects on liver, muscle and adipose tissue.
▶ Complications → diabetic ketoacidosis, nephropathy, retinopathy and neuropathy.
▶ Keep on checking the parents' understanding, provide written information and offer a follow-up appointment.

Your notes:

This is a 9-minute station consisting of spoken interaction. You will have up to 2 minutes before the start of the station to read this sheet and prepare yourself. You may make notes on the paper provided.

When the bell sounds you will be invited into the examination room. Please take this instruction sheet with you. The examiner will not ask questions during the 9 minutes, but will warn you when you have approximately 2 minutes left.

You are not required to examine a patient.

The encounter should be focused on the task: you will be penalised for asking irrelevant questions or providing superfluous information. You will be marked on your ability to communicate, not the speed with which you convey information. You may not have time to complete the communication.

Role: Paediatric registrar.

Setting: Children's outpatient clinic of a large DGH.

You are talking to: Lucy and her parents, Mr and Mrs Everington.

Background information: Lucy is a 13½-year-old girl who has been seen in the endocrine clinic with concerns regarding short stature and delayed puberty. She has had a battery of investigations, and the karyotype revealed that she has Turner's syndrome.

The diagnosis was explained to Lucy and her parents last week when they were in clinic. Lucy was very upset and distressed at such a diagnosis. Her parents were very supportive and tried to reassure Lucy. They have returned today for further explanation of her condition, as they felt that they did not take in any information on the day the diagnosis was explained to them, due to Lucy's level of distress.

Task: Please discuss with Lucy and her parents the diagnosis of Turner's syndrome.

Points to consider:

▶ Thank the family for coming back to meet with you today.
▶ First establish what information they were given at the last visit, and how much of it they can remember.

▶ The most likely situation is that they can actually remember very little, so offer to go back to the beginning, and invite them to stop you if the information is too basic.

▶ Give the basic information as follows.

▶ Chromosomes 45XO.

▶ Incidence around 1 in 2500.

▶ May be picked up at birth: carpal or pedal oedema, hypoplastic nails, feeding difficulties, short stature.

▶ Phenotype in older children: short stature, delayed puberty, webbing of the neck, low hairline, widely spaced hypoplastic nipples, increased carrying angle of the arms.

▶ There may be problems with:
  — cardiac defects – coarctation of the aorta
  — mental abilities – visuo-spatial awareness
  — hearing defects – secretary otitis media
  — fertility – ovarian dysgenesis
  — other – renal/thyroid abnormalities.

▶ After each section, pause and confirm their understanding.

▶ Explain that you will arrange for Lucy to receive specialist advice (cardiac, endocrine, etc.).

▶ Briefly discuss treatment. Often the family's main concerns will be growth and fertility.

▶ When bringing the discussion to a close, consider raising the following issues:
  — meeting other families/young people with Turner's syndrome
  — Turner's syndrome support groups
  — Internet resources/written information
  — offer to talk with Lucy and/or her parents alone.

Your notes:

This is a 9-minute station consisting of spoken interaction. You will have up to 2 minutes before the start of the station to read this sheet and prepare yourself. You may make notes on the paper provided.

When the bell sounds you will be invited into the examination room. Please take this instruction sheet with you. The examiner will not ask questions during the 9 minutes, but will warn you when you have approximately 2 minutes left.

You are not required to examine a patient.

The encounter should be focused on the task: you will be penalised for asking irrelevant questions or providing superfluous information. You will be marked on your ability to communicate, not the speed with which you convey information. You may not have time to complete the communication.

Role: Paediatric specialist registrar.

Setting: Paediatric ward in a DGH.

You are talking to: Louise, a 14-year-old girl who has been admitted with a probable diagnosis of acute lymphoblastic leukaemia (ALL).

Background information: Louise has been unwell for 6 to 8 weeks with a history of lethargy, easy bruising and shortness of breath. She has seen her general practitioner on a number of occasions, and they arranged her admission to the paediatric day unit. Arrangements have been made to transfer Louise to the tertiary oncology unit later today, where she will have a bone-marrow aspiration. Louise has asked to speak to you about the procedure. Her mother has gone home to collect some clothes for her.

Task: Talk to Louise, explaining the procedure and addressing any concerns that she may have.

Points to consider:

▶ Ask her what she understands about her illness and the proposed procedure.
▶ Explain that she will have a chance to go over the procedure in more detail with the doctor at the tertiary centre.

▶ Does she know what 'bone marrow' is?

▶ Bone marrow is the place in your body where blood cells are made. When old cells are removed, new ones are made. Sometimes things go wrong and we need to take a sample to find out what is causing the problem.

▶ We take a sample to look at the cells under the microscope. This also helps us to decide what is the best treatment for you.

▶ Explain about the procedure: general anaesthetic, use of EMLA (local anaesthetic cream).

▶ Using a special needle, we take a sample from the iliac crest (usually). Show her the area over the hip.

▶ Pain relief is provided post-operatively. Often stiff but usually well tolerated.

▶ Ask her whether she has any specific worries.

▶ Does she understand what you have said?

▶ Finally, summarise what you have told her, and offer written information and diagrams.

Your notes:

This is a 9-minute station consisting of spoken interaction. You will have up to 2 minutes before the start of the station to read this sheet and prepare yourself. You may make notes on the paper provided.

When the bell sounds you will be invited into the examination room. Please take this instruction sheet with you. The examiner will not ask questions during the 9 minutes, but will warn you when you have approximately 2 minutes left.

You are not required to examine a patient.

The encounter should be focused on the task: you will be penalised for asking irrelevant questions or providing superfluous information. You will be marked on your ability to communicate, not the speed with which you convey information. You may not have time to complete the communication.

Role: Neonatal registrar working in a busy tertiary unit.

Setting: Side room in the antenatal clinic.

You are talking to: Mrs Simpkins.

Background information: Mrs Simpkins is a 34-year-old woman who is 28 weeks pregnant with her first child. She is known to be HIV positive. The obstetric team have asked you to talk to her about what this will entail for her baby.

Task: Please talk to Mrs Simpkins and explain the implications that her condition has for her unborn child and outline the future management.

Points to consider:

▶ Mrs Simpkins may find this information very distressing, and you should acknowledge this from the outset.
▶ Consider breaking this conversation down into small chunks. Using clear signposting will help you and her to focus on the information you are giving.
— What is her understanding of HIV/AIDS?
— What is her health like at present? Is she well?
— What medication is she on?

— Explain how children become infected with HIV.
— Current recommendations, including those with regard to pregnancy, delivery, feeding, immunisations and treatment.
— Explain how HIV is diagnosed in babies.
— Prophylaxis.
▶ If appropriate, offer written information, advice about support groups, and contact telephone numbers.
▶ Confirm her understanding and arrange a follow-up appointment.

Your notes:

This is a 9-minute station consisting of spoken interaction. You will have up to 2 minutes before the start of the station to read this sheet and prepare yourself. You may make notes on the paper provided.

When the bell sounds you will be invited into the examination room. Please take this instruction sheet with you. The examiner will not ask questions during the 9 minutes, but will warn you when you have approximately 2 minutes left.

You are not required to examine a patient.

The encounter should be focused on the task: you will be penalised for asking irrelevant questions or providing superfluous information. You will be marked on your ability to communicate, not the speed with which you convey information. You may not have time to complete the communication.

Role: Paediatric specialist registrar working on the children's ward in a DGH.

Setting: Side room of the children's ward.

You are talking to: Mrs Mulholland, mother of 5-year-old Harry.

Background information: Harry is a 5-year-old asthmatic. He was admitted to your ward 2 days ago with his third exacerbation of asthma. He is receiving a course of oral steroids and is nearly ready for discharge home. After discussing him with your consultant, you wish to start him on prophylactic steroids. Prior to this admission Harry was receiving salbutamol via a spacer, and was using this up to four times daily. He is an otherwise healthy child, with both height and weight on the 25th centile. Harry's father was with him when you saw Harry on the ward round. He was happy to start the recommended treatment. Harry's mother has come to the ward and wants to talk to you, as she is unhappy about Harry being on steroids.

> Task: Please discuss with Mrs Mulholland the recommended treatment for Harry, and try to answer any questions she may have.

Points to consider:

- Thank Mrs Mulholland for coming to the ward to discuss Harry's asthma and management.
- Ask a general opening question about what she understands about the diagnosis of asthma.
- Explain in basic terms the two different types of inhaler (i.e. reliever and preventer).
- Harry is using a lot of his 'blue' inhaler, and his asthma would be better managed by trying to prevent his symptoms instead of treating them once they have occurred.
- Discuss known trigger factors or precipitants if this is an area of concern.
- Ask her why she is worried about the use of a steroid inhaler.
- Most parents are worried about the side-effects of steroids.
- Consider splitting your discussion of side-effects into local (e.g. oral candidaisis, sore throat) and systemic effects.
- Know your side-effects of steroids. Parents are often very knowledgeable. Growth is an important topic to discuss, but also easy bruising, cataracts, obesity, osteoporosis, and increased risk of infections.
- All of these side-effects are rare with low-dose inhaled steroids, but more common in high-dose oral steroids that are used on a regular basis.
- If it is growth that she is most concerned about, it is important to emphasise that there is no doubt that poorly controlled asthma has inhibitory effects on growth, and it is therefore difficult to separate the effects of asthma itself on growth from the side-effects of steroids.
- Reassure her that most children with asthma reach normal adult heights as predicted by parental height. Explain that Harry would be carefully monitored and that treatment would be tailored accordingly.
- Summarise what you have told her, offer written advice, and give her an opportunity to ask questions.

Your notes:

This is a 9-minute station consisting of spoken interaction. You will have up to 2 minutes before the start of the station to read this sheet and prepare yourself. You may make notes on the paper provided.

When the bell sounds you will be invited into the examination room. Please take this instruction sheet with you. The examiner will not ask questions during the 9 minutes, but will warn you when you have approximately 2 minutes left.

You are not required to examine a patient.

The encounter should be focused on the task: you will be penalised for asking irrelevant questions or providing superfluous information. You will be marked on your ability to communicate, not the speed with which you convey information. You may not have time to complete the communication.

Role: Paediatric registrar.

Setting: Outpatient department in a DGH.

You are talking to: Mrs Lancaster, mother of 2-year-old Christian.

Background information: Christian was born pre-term at 26 weeks' gestation. He had a stormy neonatal course that required prolonged periods of ventilation, and he was discharged home on nasal cannula oxygen which he required until his first birthday. Christian has cerebral palsy and epilepsy. He is fed via a nasogastric tube, and takes nothing orally. He has been referred to the paediatric surgeons at the tertiary centre for a gastrostomy, as he is becoming increasingly distressed each time a nasogastric tube is passed.

Task: Discuss the procedure of gastrostomy insertion, and identify Christian's mother's concerns about this procedure.

Points to consider:

 Ascertain Mrs Lancaster's understanding of the procedure.
 What are her main concerns?
 Ask specifically about the anaesthetic side of the procedure. Reassure her that the anaesthetic would be given by a paediatric anaesthetist in a tertiary centre.

- Does she know any other children who have a gastrostomy?
- Does she feel that the procedure will be of benefit to Christian?
- Remember that different centres will perform open surgery vs. percutaneous endoscopic gastrostomy (PEG).
- Most children tolerate the procedure very well, with good pain control postoperatively.
- The procedure will significantly reduce Christian's level of distress when he is being fed.
- Models are available which make explaining the procedure much easier, and you can practise changing the tube.
- Offer to arrange a time to meet with the gastrostomy liaison nurse.
- Ensure that written information, with diagrams, is available.
- Finally, ask Mrs Lancaster whether she has any further questions, and offer a repeat appointment if she still has unanswered questions or further concerns.

Your notes:

••

This is a 9-minute station consisting of spoken interaction. You will have up to 2 minutes before the start of the station to read this sheet and prepare yourself. You may make notes on the paper provided.

When the bell sounds you will be invited into the examination room. Please take this instruction sheet with you. The examiner will not ask questions during the 9 minutes, but will warn you when you have approximately 2 minutes left.

You are not required to examine a patient.

The encounter should be focused on the task: you will be penalised for asking irrelevant questions or providing superfluous information. You will be marked on your ability to communicate, not the speed with which you convey information. You may not have time to complete the communication.

••

Role: Paediatric registrar, working in a busy DGH.

Setting: Side room in the children's outpatient department.

You are talking to: Mr and Mrs Fitzgerald, parents of 3-year-old John.

Background information: John is a 3-year-old boy who has Duchenne muscular dystrophy. He has just attended your clinic for outpatient follow-up. He is also seen by the muscle team in the tertiary unit. At the end of their clinic appointment, John's parents ask whether you could discuss the implications of John's condition for any future pregnancy.

Task: John's parents are considering having a second child. Please discuss the implications of John's diagnosis with regard to any future pregnancies.

Points to consider:

▶ Clarify John's parents' reason for wanting to see you, so that there can be no misunderstandings.
▶ What do they understand of the inheritance pattern of Duchenne muscular dystrophy?
▶ Outline the basic genetics:
  — X-linked recessive condition
  — one-third of cases are new mutations

    — female carriers are usually asymptomatic

    — the condition is due to mutations in the dystrophin gene.

▶ Chances of an affected pregnancy:

    — 25% risk of an affected male (if the mother is a carrier)

    — 25% risk of a carrier female.

▶ Antenatal diagnosis – if appropriate, mention termination of pregnancy.

▶ Diagnosis of live-born infant:

    — muscle biopsy

    — raised plasma creatine kinase

    — mutations in dystrophin gene.

▶ Point out that you have given them a great deal of information on a difficult topic. You are not a geneticist, and you feel that it would be appropriate for them to be referred if they would like the opportunity for this.

▶ Offer written information, a genetics referral and a follow-up appointment.

Your notes:

This is a 9-minute station consisting of spoken interaction. You will have up to 2 minutes before the start of the station to read this sheet and prepare yourself. You may make notes on the paper provided.

When the bell sounds you will be invited into the examination room. Please take this instruction sheet with you. The examiner will not ask questions during the 9 minutes, but will warn you when you have approximately 2 minutes left.

You are not required to examine a patient.

The encounter should be focused on the task: you will be penalised for asking irrelevant questions or providing superfluous information. You will be marked on your ability to communicate, not the speed with which you convey information. You may not have time to complete the communication.

Role: Neonatal registrar working in a busy tertiary unit.

Setting: Side room on the antenatal ward.

You are talking to: Melanie Anderson, a 25-year-old single mother.

Background information: Melanie is 26 weeks' pregnant with her second child. She has been given antenatal steroids as she is in early labour. The obstetricians think it is very likely that she will deliver within the next 24 hours, and have asked you to talk to her prior to the onset of established labour.

Task: Please talk to Melanie about preterm babies, and discuss some of the difficulties and complications they are likely to encounter. Try to answer any other questions that she may have.

Points to consider:

▶ Introduce yourself, and ask Melanie whether she has a partner, friend or relative whom she would like to be present.
▶ Explain why you have been asked to come and talk to her, and what your role would be once the baby is born.
▶ Does she know any babies who have been born very early? Does she know much about the problems they can face?
▶ You need to be clear that some babies who are born this early

are, despite everything we do to help them, not strong enough to survive. Those who do survive have a very lengthy stay in hospital (as a rough guide, until they get to term). There will be a number of problems/complications during this period.

▶ All such extreme preterm babies will need help to stabilise them at birth, and will require subsequent care on the intensive-care unit. The parents may wish to visit the neonatal unit and meet the staff.

▶ Explain exactly who will be present when the baby is born – the obstetric team, the neonatal team and the mother's midwife – explaining the role of each.

▶ Consider taking Melanie through this in a very structured manner. It may be more appropriate to start with immediate problems (stiff lungs, surfactant treatment, need for support on a breathing machine, oxygen), and to reassure her that other issues will be discussed and/or dealt with as they present. The parents will have ample opportunities to meet up with the medical team on a regular basis.

— Respiratory problems, including surfactant treatment, intubation and ventilation, CPAP, home oxygen.

— Cardiovascular problems: possible PDA, need for inotropes, blood pressure stabilisation.

— Gut problems: immature bowel, TPN, formula or expressed breast milk, necrotising enterocolitis.

— Neurological problems: intra-ventricular haemorrhages, seizures, hydrocephalus, adverse neurodevelopment.

— Eye problems: retinopathy of prematurity.

— Other: temperature control, infection, vascular access, chronic lung disease.

▶ Acknowledge that this is a vast amount of information.

▶ Explain that the baby will be cared for in the neonatal unit, and as soon as Melanie is feeling well enough after delivery she would be able to visit her baby.

▶ Arrange a second meeting so that she has time to think about what you have told her and ask any further questions.

Your notes:

This is a 9-minute station consisting of spoken interaction. You will have up to 2 minutes before the start of the station to read this sheet and prepare yourself. You may make notes on the paper provided.

When the bell sounds you will be invited into the examination room. Please take this instruction sheet with you. The examiner will not ask questions during the 9 minutes, but will warn you when you have approximately 2 minutes left.

You are not required to examine a patient.

The encounter should be focused on the task: you will be penalised for asking irrelevant questions or providing superfluous information. You will be marked on your ability to communicate, not the speed with which you convey information. You may not have time to complete the communication.

Role: Paediatric registrar working in a busy DGH.

Setting: Clinic room in the outpatient department.

You are talking to: Mrs Barwick, mother of 7-year-old Edwin.

Background information: Edwin is a 7-year-old boy who has a diagnosis of hereditary spherocytosis. He is seen regularly by the haematologist and the paediatric team. Due to recurrent haemolysis, he is going to have a splenectomy under the care of the paediatric surgeons in 2 weeks' time. He is an otherwise healthy child. Mrs Barwick has given consent for surgery, but remains worried about the consequences, and has asked for a further appointment to meet you prior to the planned surgery.

Task: Please talk to Edwin's mother and try to address her concerns with regard to Edwin's diagnosis and forthcoming splenectomy.

Points to consider:

▶ Begin by establishing Mrs Barwick's current understanding of Edwin's diagnosis of hereditary spherocytosis (HS).
▶ Does she have any specific questions or worries? If not, one way to tackle this may be to go through things in basic terms.

- Go back to basics, and explain the function of the spleen. It is a large organ on the left-hand side of the body, below and behind the stomach. One of its main functions is to remove worn out red blood cells and other foreign bodies from the bloodstream. In hereditary spherocytosis, the red blood cells have a fragile membrane and are therefore removed at a faster rate by the spleen.
- Explain the consequences of HS. These include anaemia (i.e. low haemoglobin), intermittent jaundice and chronic haemolysis (breakdown of blood cells)), which can lead to the formation of gallstones. All of these can be precipitated by a viral infection, and one possible complication is aplastic anaemia.
- Discuss the benefits of Edwin having a splenectomy. It will decrease the rate of destruction of the red blood cells, and will also lower the possibility of traumatic rupture of the spleen.
- Discuss the risks of the procedure. Overwhelming sepsis (infection) is due to the function of the spleen in dealing with encapsulated organisms. We can minimise this risk, so that now the benefits out-weigh the risks. If possible, delay the surgery until after 5 years of age, and ensure an adequate level of vaccinations, including pneumovax and Hib. Prophylactic penicillin V will be needed for life.
- Advise the use of a Medic-alert bracelet, and tell Mrs Barwick to seek urgent medical attention if Edwin is unwell.
- The actual surgery will be explained in further detail by the surgeon who will be performing the operation.
- Ask whether this information has answered her questions, whether it has reassured her, and whether she has any further questions.
- If necessary, arrange a further meeting, and provide written information.

Your notes:

This is a 9-minute station consisting of spoken interaction. You will have up to 2 minutes before the start of the station to read this sheet and prepare yourself. You may make notes on the paper provided.

When the bell sounds you will be invited into the examination room. Please take this instruction sheet with you. The examiner will not ask questions during the 9 minutes, but will warn you when you have approximately 2 minutes left.

You are not required to examine a patient.

The encounter should be focused on the task: you will be penalised for asking irrelevant questions or providing superfluous information. You will be marked on your ability to communicate, not the speed with which you convey information. You may not have time to complete the communication.

Role: Paediatric specialist registrar.

Setting: Outpatient clinic.

You are talking to: Mr Jenkins, father of 18-month-old Holly.

Background information: Holly has primary ciliary dyskinesia, and although her general health is good, she suffers from recurrent chest infections which require prolonged stays in hospital for IV antibiotic therapy. IV access is always difficult, and it is becoming more distressing for both Holly and her parents each time she is admitted to hospital. At the last clinic appointment the possibility of port insertion was raised with her parents, and they have returned today to explore this option further.

Task: Discuss with Mr Jenkins the advantages and disadvantages of Portacath insertion for his daughter, and try to answer any questions he may have.

Points to consider:

▶ Explain that you are happy to talk to Mr Jenkins about Portacath insertion. However, if the parents decide to go ahead with the procedure, they would have the opportunity to discuss the procedure in greater detail with the surgeon who would be performing the operation.

- What is Mr Jenkin's understanding of what a Portacath is and does?
- How does he feel a port will benefit Holly?
- Does he think that there are any disadvantages?
- The procedure will require a general anaesthetic.
- The cosmetic side of things may not be a concern now while Holly is small, but may become an issue as she enters her teenage years. How will they address this?
- Does he know of any other children who have ports?
- There are mannequins available to demonstrate ports and Hickman lines. Offer to arrange to show him one at a later date.
- You can either refer him to the paediatric surgeons or, if he feels that he needs longer to think about it, you can meet him again, possibly with Holly's mother.

Your notes:

This is a 9-minute station consisting of spoken interaction. You will have up to 2 minutes before the start of the station to read this sheet and prepare yourself. You may make notes on the paper provided.

When the bell sounds you will be invited into the examination room. Please take this instruction sheet with you. The examiner will not ask questions during the 9 minutes, but will warn you when you have approximately 2 minutes left.

You are not required to examine a patient.

The encounter should be focused on the task: you will be penalised for asking irrelevant questions or providing superfluous information. You will be marked on your ability to communicate, not the speed with which you convey information. You may not have time to complete the communication.

Role: Paediatric specialist registrar.

Setting: Side room of the paediatric day unit in a DGH.

You are talking to: Mr and Mrs Jacobson, parents of 3-week-old Bethany.

Background information: Bethany was born at term after an uncomplicated pregnancy, and required no resuscitation at birth. She has struggled to open her bowels since birth, and on further questioning you find out that she did not pass meconium within the first 24 hours of life. Your consultant has reviewed Bethany on a number of occasions. After discussion with the surgical team, it was decided to perform a rectal biopsy the following day to exclude a diagnosis of Hirschsprung's disease.

Task: Your consultant has explained to Bethany's parents the need for a rectal biopsy, but now has to go to clinic, and has asked you to have a further discussion with them and to explain the procedure.

Points to consider:

▶ What are the parents' thoughts about why Bethany is having such difficulty opening her bowels?
▶ Does anyone else in the family have similar problems?

▮ Do the parents understand why you are going to do a rectal biopsy?

▮ Explain briefly what the procedure involves. Three small samples of tissue will be taken from the back passage in order to look at the cells under the microscope.

▮ The procedure does not usually require a general anaesthetic. It is possible to use sucrose (sugar) orally in small babies for pain relief.

▮ It is a short procedure, well tolerated by most babies.

▮ The parents can feed, bathe and comfort Bethany as they usually do.

▮ What is the intended aim of the biopsy (i.e. to confirm/exclude Hirschsprung's disease)?

▮ Do not go into great detail about Hirschsprung's disease. Give a brief explanation, and then mention that if necessary you will spend some time going over the condition in more detail.

▮ Do the parents have any particular concerns?

Your notes:

This is a 9-minute station consisting of spoken interaction. You will have up to 2 minutes before the start of the station to read this sheet and prepare yourself. You may make notes on the paper provided.

When the bell sounds you will be invited into the examination room. Please take this instruction sheet with you. The examiner will not ask questions during the 9 minutes, but will warn you when you have approximately 2 minutes left.

You are not required to examine a patient.

The encounter should be focused on the task: you will be penalised for asking irrelevant questions or providing superfluous information. You will be marked on your ability to communicate, not the speed with which you convey information. You may not have time to complete the communication.

Role: Paediatric specialist registrar.

Setting: The relatives' room on a children's ward.

You are talking to: Mrs Maggie Stephens, mother of 5-year-old Sadie.

Background information: Sadie is a 5-year-old girl with severe cerebral palsy. She is currently an inpatient on your ward. She was admitted 10 days ago with a chest infection, and this is her fourth admission this year, each time presenting with a chest infection. She has suffered from gastro-oesophageal reflux for a number of years. She is fed via a nasogastric tube. Her parents have resisted the idea of fundoplication for a long time, and have persisted with medical and conservative management of her reflux. During this admission she has had a pH study and further imaging, as well as being assessed by the physiotherapist and speech and language therapist. Her recurrent chest infections are thought to be caused by aspiration.

Task: You have been asked by your consultant to re-explore the idea of fundoplication with Sadie's mother.

Points to consider:

▶ Introduce the idea that you would like to talk to Sadie's mother about the possibility of Sadie having a fundoplication.

▶ Make it clear that you understand that she has not been keen on the idea in the past, but you wondered if it would be all right with her if you could talk to her.

▶ Explain why you as a medical team feel that the procedure is in Sadie's best interests, as there is a constant risk of aspiration, and Sadie's chest infections are becoming more severe.

▶ Also during this admission you needed to use alternative antibiotics due to resistant bacteria, and this is due to the repeated courses of treatment.

▶ Listen to Sadie's mother's concerns, be empathic, and let her explain why she is not keen to go ahead.

▶ Offer to briefly describe the procedure, and draw a diagram, as this makes it much easier to visualise.

▶ Sadie's mother may have specific concerns regarding the general anaesthetic, and the increased risk associated with an anaesthetic in children like Sadie.

▶ Provide her with some written information, give her time and space, and do not pressurise her.

▶ Offer to meet again once she has had time to think about what has been said. You understand that it is a difficult decision to make, and are happy to try to answer any further questions that she and her husband may have.

Your notes:

This is a 9-minute station consisting of spoken interaction. You will have up to 2 minutes before the start of the station to read this sheet and prepare yourself. You may make notes on the paper provided.

When the bell sounds you will be invited into the examination room. Please take this instruction sheet with you. The examiner will not ask questions during the 9 minutes, but will warn you when you have approximately 2 minutes left.

You are not required to examine a patient.

The encounter should be focused on the task: you will be penalised for asking irrelevant questions or providing superfluous information. You will be marked on your ability to communicate, not the speed with which you convey information. You may not have time to complete the communication.

Role: Paediatric specialist registrar.

Setting: Paediatric outpatient department.

You are talking to: Marcus, a 15-year-old boy.

Background information: Marcus was first referred to the paediatric department 4 months ago. He has a long history of lethargy and fatigue which seemed to follow a viral upper respiratory tract infection. He complains of severe headaches, for which he had an MRI scan, which is reported as normal. He has been fully investigated, and all of the findings are normal. A diagnosis of chronic fatigue syndrome has been made. Marcus has returned to clinic today with his parents, but has asked to have the consultation alone.

Task: Explain to Marcus the diagnosis of chronic fatigue syndrome and the subsequent management of the condition.

Points to consider:

▶ Find out what Marcus thinks about his symptoms, and what he feels is causing his symptoms.

▶ Giving children and young people the opportunity to voice their concerns will often reveal their underlying anxieties.

▶ Marcus may be worried that he has a brain tumour. Only when you have explored his concerns will you be able to provide reassurance.

▶ Talk about the diagnosis and what this means for him.

▶ In terms of management, different centres will have different approaches, but consider psychological input, and assistance from a physiotherapist and an occupational therapist.

▶ Discuss educational involvement and a graded exercise programme tailored to his specific needs.

▶ Most important is the need for a multi-disciplinary team approach, with the paediatrician acting as team coordinator.

▶ You can reassure Marcus that although little is known about this condition, young people like him often do very well with a structured programme.

▶ Offer follow-up and written information.

▶ Clarify his understanding and ask whether there is anything else that he wishes to discuss with you.

Your notes:

This is a 9-minute station consisting of spoken interaction. You will have up to 2 minutes before the start of the station to read this sheet and prepare yourself. You may make notes on the paper provided.

When the bell sounds you will be invited into the examination room. Please take this instruction sheet with you. The examiner will not ask questions during the 9 minutes, but will warn you when you have approximately 2 minutes left.

You are not required to examine a patient.

The encounter should be focused on the task: you will be penalised for asking irrelevant questions or providing superfluous information. You will be marked on your ability to communicate, not the speed with which you convey information. You may not have time to complete the communication.

Role: Paediatric registrar.

Setting: Outpatient clinic in a busy DGH.

You are talking to: Jamie, a 15-year-old boy.

Background information: Jamie was diagnosed with myoclonic epilepsy about 18 months ago. An EEG has confirmed the diagnosis, and an MRI brain scan was normal. His seizures are now well controlled using sodium valproate. Jamie attends clinic regularly accompanied by his mother or father, and is compliant with treatment. He is doing well academically. He has no other medical problems. Jamie has attended clinic today with his mother, but at the end of the consultation has asked to speak to you alone.

Task: Please talk to Jamie and find out what he wishes to discuss with you, trying to answer any questions he may have.

Points to consider:

▶ Start the consultation by asking how Jamie is getting on. There may be issues that he wants to discuss, but he feels uncomfortable about doing so in the presence of his mother.
▶ Try to address any specific concerns that he has.
▶ Another way to structure the consultation would be to take things

back to a basic level. What does he understand by the diagnosis of epilepsy?

▶ Epilepsy is when the signals in your brain get mixed up and too much electrical activity is discharged at once. When this happens you have a fit or seizure.

▶ There are many different types of epilepsy. He has something called 'myoclonic epilepsy', which can be described as brief, sudden, generalised movements of the arms, legs, neck and trunk.

▶ It is common, occurring in about 5 in 1000 school-age children.

▶ In most people we do not know the exact underlying cause of their fits. This is called idiopathic epilepsy.

▶ We can do different investigations to help us. An EEG looks at the electrical activity inside the brain. Draw a diagram to illustrate a normal EEG wave pattern and an abnormal pattern.

▶ Jamie's seizures are controlled using anti-epileptic medication. Does he experience any side-effects (increased appetite, weight gain, hair loss)?

▶ Sometimes certain factors can trigger a fit, such as lack of sleep, alcohol, drugs, excitement or anxiety. At this point you can ask specifically whether he has any concerns about any of these issues.

▶ Acknowledge that this is a difficult time for him, due to the changes of puberty, as well as peer pressure.

▶ Ask about friendships and school (and sexual relationships if you feel this is appropriate).

▶ Clarify that you have covered all of the areas of concern. Ask if there is anything else you can help him with. Assure him that you would be happy to see him again if necessary.

▶ Offer him contact telephone numbers and details of support groups. Suggest that perhaps meeting other young people with epilepsy may be of benefit.

Your notes:

This is a 9-minute station consisting of spoken interaction. You will have up to 2 minutes before the start of the station to read this sheet and prepare yourself. You may make notes on the paper provided.

When the bell sounds you will be invited into the examination room. Please take this instruction sheet with you. The examiner will not ask questions during the 9 minutes, but will warn you when you have approximately 2 minutes left.

You are not required to examine a patient.

The encounter should be focused on the task: you will be penalised for asking irrelevant questions or providing superfluous information. You will be marked on your ability to communicate, not the speed with which you convey information. You may not have time to complete the communication.

Role: Paediatric specialist registrar.

Setting: Outpatient clinic in a DGH.

You are talking to: Mr and Mrs Jessop and their 6-year-old daughter Rosie.

Background information: Rosie is a 6-year-old girl who has been seen by the paediatric rheumatologist at the tertiary hospital. She has been diagnosed with oligoarticular juvenile idiopathic arthritis. A follow-up appointment in 4 weeks' time has been arranged.

Task: Please discuss with Rosie's parents what the diagnosis means in terms of prognosis, management and treatment. You may try to answer any other questions they may have.

Points to consider:

▶ Clarify their understanding of juvenile idiopathic arthritis:
— juvenile = child
— idiopathic = exact cause is not known
— arthritis = inflammation of joints.
▶ It is an inflammatory process, and the aim is to decrease inflammation and maintain remission.
▶ Treatment: steroids (oral, IV or intra-articular).

▶ At this point you can mention that many parents are concerned about side-effects, which include growth, obesity, thinning skin, bruising, osteoporosis and cushingoid facies.

▶ Other treatments available: NSAIDs and methotrexate.

▶ Management: multi-disciplinary team including doctors, nurses, physiotherapists, occupational therapists and education.

▶ Distribution: approximately 10% systemic, 60% oligoarticular and 30% polyarticular.

▶ Prognosis: as a rough guide, a third of children will get better with no residual symptoms, a third will improve but will have residual symptoms, and the remaining third will deteriorate. Children with the oligoarticular type generally have a better outcome.

▶ Offer further appointments if Rosie's parents still have outstanding questions or concerns. If they ask questions to which you are not sure of the answer, offer to research this, speak with the tertiary hospital and get back to them.

▶ You could also mention support groups.

Your notes:

This is a 9-minute station consisting of spoken interaction. You will have up to 2 minutes before the start of the station to read this sheet and prepare yourself. You may make notes on the paper provided.

When the bell sounds you will be invited into the examination room. Please take this instruction sheet with you. The examiner will not ask questions during the 9 minutes, but will warn you when you have approximately 2 minutes left.

You are not required to examine a patient.

The encounter should be focused on the task: you will be penalised for asking irrelevant questions or providing superfluous information. You will be marked on your ability to communicate, not the speed with which you convey information. You may not have time to complete the communication.

Role: Paediatric registrar working in a busy DGH.

Setting: Children's outpatient department.

You are talking to: Mrs Harris, mother of 11-month-old Oliver.

Background information: Oliver has been attending your clinic over the last 4 months, undergoing investigations for neurofibromatosis type 1. His father also has the condition.

Oliver has been seen this morning by the tertiary genetics team, who have confirmed the diagnosis. His mother has asked if you could explain the diagnosis again to her, as although her husband has the condition, she has never really understood what it means.

Task: Please explain the diagnosis of neurofibromatosis type 1 to Mrs Harris.

Points to consider:

 First establish her background level of knowledge, as this will give you a starting point.

 Explain that neurofibromatosis type 1 is the most common of the neurocutaneous syndromes. You will need to explain what you mean by the term 'neurocutaneous.'

 Then try to go through the condition in a structured format:

  — genetics/inheritance
  — clinical diagnosis (i.e. here you should know that the diagnosis
     is made by fulfilling two or more of the six main criteria, and be
     able to list these criteria)
  — associated clinical findings and complications
  — management and treatment
  — follow-up and prognosis.
▶ Confirm Mrs Harris's understanding, and answer any questions
  that she may have.
▶ There is an excellent website on neurofibromatosis to which you
  could direct her for further information: www.nfauk.org/nfauk_
  downloads/nf1-factsheets/introduction_to_nf-info_for_families.pdf
▶ Provide written information and arrange follow-up.

Note: The diagnostic criteria and associated complications are available
in standard paediatric texts.

Your notes:

. . . .

This is a 9-minute station consisting of spoken interaction. You will have up to 2 minutes before the start of the station to read this sheet and prepare yourself. You may make notes on the paper provided.

When the bell sounds you will be invited into the examination room. Please take this instruction sheet with you. The examiner will not ask questions during the 9 minutes, but will warn you when you have approximately 2 minutes left.

You are not required to examine a patient.

The encounter should be focused on the task: you will be penalised for asking irrelevant questions or providing superfluous information. You will be marked on your ability to communicate, not the speed with which you convey information. You may not have time to complete the communication.

. . . .

Role: Paediatric registrar working on the day unit in a busy DGH.

Setting: Side room of the day unit.

You are talking to: Mrs Leigh, mother of 8-month-old Thomas.

Background information: Thomas was born at term after an uneventful pregnancy. He has been well until 2 days ago, when he presented to the day unit with a history of temperature and vomiting. Urine dipstick and microscopy have confirmed the diagnosis of urinary tract infection. He is clinically well hydrated, and his temperature has come down since he has been given paracetamol. His weight, height and head circumference are all on the 50th centile, and his development is age appropriate.

Task: Please inform Thomas's mother of the diagnosis of urinary tract infection, and explain that Thomas will require both a treatment course and prophylactic antibiotics. He will also need a renal USS, DMSA scan and MCUG. Try to address any other concerns that Mrs Leigh may have.

Points to consider:

▶ Use a simple diagram to explain the diagnosis.
▶ Go through each area of treatment and investigations in a structured manner.

▶ Always refer to individual unit protocols, and be aware of the new NICE guidelines. If you are unsure, you can always say that you will explain the management and then confirm this with your consultant.

▶ Adopt a clear approach: first a treatment course of antibiotics, and then change to prophylactic antibiotics. You should highlight the need to continue this until all the scans have been completed, and if negative they will be advised to stop treatment.

▶ Explain the need for the three investigations, and discuss briefly what each one entails:

1 renal USS – this is used to identify any structural abnormalities, and to assess the shape, position and size of each kidney

2 DMSA scan – this requires an injection of dye in order to determine whether there is any damage to the kidney, which would show up as a scar; it is also used to assess the functioning of each kidney

3 MCUG – in this procedure a tube is inserted into the bladder (use your diagram to illustrate this), to determine whether any urine goes back up the wrong way into the kidneys (i.e. reflux).

▶ Explain why each of these investigations is important, the aim being to prevent further infections, kidney damage and end-stage renal failure.

▶ This is a lot of information to deliver at one sitting. However, if they are given clear diagrams and written information leaflets, parents usually gain a clear understanding.

▶ Confirm Mrs Leigh's understanding by asking her to repeat the information back to you, and arrange follow-up as appropriate.

Your notes:

This is a 9-minute station consisting of spoken interaction. You will have up to 2 minutes before the start of the station to read this sheet and prepare yourself. You may make notes on the paper provided.

When the bell sounds you will be invited into the examination room. Please take this instruction sheet with you. The examiner will not ask questions during the 9 minutes, but will warn you when you have approximately 2 minutes left.

You are not required to examine a patient.

The encounter should be focused on the task: you will be penalised for asking irrelevant questions or providing superfluous information. You will be marked on your ability to communicate, not the speed with which you convey information. You may not have time to complete the communication.

Role: Neonatal registrar working in a busy DGH.

Setting: Side room on the postnatal ward.

You are talking to: Mrs Roberts, mother of baby Sophie, who is now 24 hours old.

Background information: Sophie was born yesterday at term, weighing 3.5 kg, after an uneventful pregnancy. She has been feeding well and is ready to be discharged home this morning. Mrs Roberts is anxious to speak to you, as her father has recently been diagnosed with Huntington's disease, and she is worried about the possible implications for Sophie.

Task: Please discuss the concerns that Mrs Roberts has raised regarding her father's recent diagnosis.

Points to consider:

▶ Congratulate Mrs Roberts on the birth of Sophie, and ask her if she would like to have a friend, relative or her partner present.
▶ Express your sympathy: 'I'm sorry to hear of your father's recent diagnosis. Had he been unwell for a long time?'
▶ Find out what she knows about Huntington's disease.
▶ Explain that you are not a geneticist but are able to give her some basic information:

— what Huntington's disease is
— how it is inherited – *autosomal dominant*
— characteristic features
— how it presents
— juvenile Huntington's disease
— diagnosis
— course and prognosis
— management.

▶ Acknowledge her main worry that baby Sophie will also have the disease. Explain that for this to have occurred, Mrs Roberts too would need to have inherited it from her father.

▶ There is a 50% chance that she has inherited the faulty gene, and a further 50% chance that she has passed it on to Sophie, giving Sophie an overall 25% risk.

▶ Summarise, and provide written information, contact telephone numbers and addresses of support groups.

▶ Offer to make a referral to a geneticist.

▶ Try to finish by again congratulating her on the birth of her daughter, and for now concentrate on her and treat her as you would any other baby.

Your notes:

This is a 9-minute station consisting of spoken interaction. You will have up to 2 minutes before the start of the station to read this sheet and prepare yourself. You may make notes on the paper provided.

When the bell sounds you will be invited into the examination room. Please take this instruction sheet with you. The examiner will not ask questions during the 9 minutes, but will warn you when you have approximately 2 minutes left.

You are not required to examine a patient.

The encounter should be focused on the task: you will be penalised for asking irrelevant questions or providing superfluous information. You will be marked on your ability to communicate, not the speed with which you convey information. You may not have time to complete the communication.

Role: Paediatric registrar working in a busy DGH.

Setting: Children's outpatient clinic.

You are talking to: Mr and Mrs Jackson, parents of 10-month-old Ryan.

Background information: Ryan is a healthy 10-month-old baby. His parents have brought him to clinic today because they are concerned about the shape of his head. Ryan has been seen by your consultant, who has diagnosed a mild form of plagiocephaly which requires no treatment. Ryan is developmentally age appropriate, and has no other medical problems.

Task: Please meet with Ryan's parents to explain the diagnosis of plagiocephaly and answer any questions they may have.

Points to consider:

▶ Explain the reason why you have been asked to meet with Ryan's parents today.
▶ What were their concerns about the shape of Ryan's head? Do they have any thoughts about what might be causing the problem?
▶ Avoiding medical jargon, explain what plagiocephaly is.
▶ This condition is likely to be of no significance, and will not affect Ryan's development in any way.

▶ Mr and Mrs Jackson may be concerned about the cosmetic appearance. and can be reassured that this improves with time.
▶ If they have researched this condition (e.g. on the Internet), they may raise other issues:
   — association with congenital syndromes – Apert's or Crouzon's syndrome
   — the wearing of a special helmet to help to remould the head
   — the use of a certain kind of mattress to mould to the shape of the baby's head.
      Neither of the latter two approaches is currently recommended by the Royal College of Paediatricians.
▶ The parents can be reassured, and you can offer further written information.
▶ If they are very anxious and difficult to reassure, offer a follow-up appointment to monitor Ryan's progress.

Your notes:

This is a 9-minute station consisting of spoken interaction. You will have up to 2 minutes before the start of the station to read this sheet and prepare yourself. You may make notes on the paper provided.

When the bell sounds you will be invited into the examination room. Please take this instruction sheet with you. The examiner will not ask questions during the 9 minutes, but will warn you when you have approximately 2 minutes left.

You are not required to examine a patient.

The encounter should be focused on the task: you will be penalised for asking irrelevant questions or providing superfluous information. You will be marked on your ability to communicate, not the speed with which you convey information. You may not have time to complete the communication.

Role: Paediatric registrar working in a busy DGH.

Setting: Side room in the children's outpatient department.

You are talking to: Emily, a 15-year-old girl who has recently been diagnosed with Crohn's disease.

Background information: Emily has been under the care of the paediatric department for the last 6 months following complaints of weight loss, altered bowel habit, fatigue and mouth ulcers. She has been fully investigated, and a diagnosis of Crohn's disease has been made. She has asked to speak to you while her parents are talking to the consultant, as she does not fully understand what the diagnosis means.

Task: Please meet with Emily, explain to her what Crohn's disease is, and try to answer any other questions she may have.

Points to consider:

▶ First clarify what she knows or understands about Crohn's disease.
▶ Start with the basics, trying to structure your conversation under sub-headings as follows:
— What is Crohn's disease?
— What investigations has she had (blood, radiological, endoscopic

procedures)? She will have had some of these tests performed, so clarify the results as you talk about each test.
— Management – pharmacological, surgical and nutritional.
— Remission – she may in particular want to discuss steroids, as this is often an area of concern for patients.
— Long-term prognosis.
▶ Does she have any other questions or concerns? Is there anything in particular that she wishes to discuss today?
▶ Offer written information, and the contact telephone numbers and addresses of support groups. Suggest that she considers meeting other young people with inflammatory bowel disease.
▶ Arrange follow-up, and offer to meet again if she would find this helpful.

Your notes:

··

This is a 6-minute station. You will have 3 minutes beforehand to read this sheet and prepare yourself. You may take the sheet with you into the station, but you must return it at the end.

··

Role: A GP registrar.

Setting: GP surgery.

You are talking to: Leigh Bailey.

Background information: Leigh is a 15-year-old girl who has had an 18-year-old boyfriend for one year and has no knowledge of contraception. She has a normal menstrual history. They have not used a condom, and Leigh finds it very difficult to discuss these issues with her boyfriend. She worries about getting pregnant and is afraid of her parents' reaction. She also demands that you do not tell her parents about this consultation.

Task: To discuss the issues relating to contraception and safe sex.

YOU ARE NOT EXPECTED TO GATHER THE REST OF THE MEDICAL HISTORY DURING THIS CONSULTATION

Points to consider:

- Try to explore and understand Leigh's anxieties about getting pregnant and her parents' reaction.
- Be comfortable discussing the issues and reassuring Leigh.
- Be non-judgmental.
- Understand her rights with regard to confidentiality.
- Explain the possibility of sexually transmitted disease and discuss safe sex.
- Arrange appropriate follow-up (family planning clinic, practice nurse, etc.).
- Check with Leigh that she has had her questions answered to her satisfaction.
- Offer to provide her with printed information about local family planning clinics.

▶ Encourage Leigh to bring her boyfriend with her for any further consultations.
▶ Encourage her to be open with her parents.

Your notes:

This is a 9-minute station consisting of spoken interaction. You will have up to 2 minutes before the start of the station to read this sheet and prepare yourself. You may make notes on the paper provided.

When the bell sounds you will be invited into the examination room. Please take this instruction sheet with you. The examiner will not ask questions during the 9 minutes, but will warn you when you have approximately 2 minutes left.

You are not required to examine a patient.

The encounter should be focused on the task: you will be penalised for asking irrelevant questions or providing superfluous information. You will be marked on your ability to communicate, not the speed with which you convey information. You may not have time to complete the communication.

Role: A paediatric specialty registrar (ST4) working in a district general hospital.

You are talking to: Bob Hagget, father of Demi, a 5-year-old girl with cystic fibrosis.

Setting: A side-room on the paediatric ward.

Background information: Demi was diagnosed with cystic fibrosis after she had meconium ileus during the early neonatal period. She was treated with anti-staphylococcal antibiotics twice daily for the first 2 years of life, and has not had troublesome respiratory symptoms until recently.

For the last 3 months she has been increasingly unwell, with tiredness and a productive cough. *Pseudomonas aeruginosa* was isolated for the first time from Demi's sputum samples taken at her last clinic appointment 2 weeks ago. She was admitted 3 days ago and is on IV ceftazidime. She also has chest physiotherapy twice a day, supervised by a paediatric physiotherapist.

Her parents separated 3 months ago, and her mother has been struggling to persuade Demi to cooperate with physiotherapy at home. There are three other children with cystic fibrosis in separate cubicles on the ward. Demi's father has come to visit her for the first time since her admission. He has questioned the nurses about the need for her admission to hospital, and is angry that she has been isolated in a cubicle.

Task: To explain to Demi's father the rationale for her current management.

YOU ARE NOT EXPECTED TO GATHER THE REST OF THE MEDICAL HISTORY DURING THIS CONSULTATION.

Points to consider:

▶ Be sensitive and sympathetic to the father's concerns and feelings.
▶ Remain non-judgmental and objective about the father's current situation.
▶ Encourage the father to express his views.
▶ Recognise the potential for the father to misinterpret the situation and to criticise Demi's mother.
▶ Ascertain the father's pre-existing knowledge of cystic fibrosis.
▶ Give a clear explanation using jargon-free language appropriate to the father's level of understanding.
▶ Avoid criticising either parent.
▶ Offer advice and further information on cystic fibrosis.
▶ Demonstrate an up-to-date knowledge of the management of cystic fibrosis.
▶ Understand the pathophysiology and treatment of *Pseudomonas aeruginosa* in children with cystic fibrosis.
▶ Clearly understand the need for isolation in a cubicle.

Your notes:

This is a 9-minute station consisting of spoken interaction. You will have up to 2 minutes before the start of the station to read this sheet and prepare yourself. You may make notes on the paper provided.

When the bell sounds you will be invited into the examination room. Please take this instruction sheet with you. The examiner will not ask questions during the 9 minutes, but will warn you when you have approximately 2 minutes left.

You are not required to examine a patient.

The encounter should be focused on the task: you will be penalised for asking irrelevant questions or providing superfluous information. You will be marked on your ability to communicate, not the speed with which you convey information. You may not have time to complete the communication.

Role: Paediatric registrar, working in a busy district general hospital.

Setting: Side-room cubicle in the A&E department.

You are talking to: Sally Jones, the mother of Daniel, who is 13 months old.

Background information: Daniel Jones has been admitted to the A&E department via his GP. He presented to the GP with symptoms of a mild upper respiratory tract infection, but on examination the GP found him to be tachycardic, with a heart rate of over 200 beats per minute. He called an ambulance to send Daniel and his mother to the A&E department.

On arrival Daniel was seen by the A&E registrar in the resuscitation room. His heart rate was 280 beats per minute. The cardiac monitor and ECG trace showed a narrow complex tachycardia, and he was treated according to Advanced Paediatric Life Support (APLS) guidelines. After receiving one dose of adenosine, Daniel's heart rhythm converted to sinus rhythm. The paediatric registrar was called to take over Daniel's management. Daniel is haemodynamically stable and his ECG now shows evidence of Wolff–Parkinson–White syndrome.

Task: To meet with Mrs Jones to explain Daniel's diagnosis and your plans for his further management, and to answer any questions that she may have.

Points to consider:

▶ Introduce yourself to the mother and explain why you have been asked to talk to her.

▶ Offer her reassurance, emphasising that Daniel is now well and stable.

▶ Elicit her concerns and understanding so far, and demonstrate empathy.

▶ Explain the diagnosis and the acute management of the condition.

▶ Explain why Wolff–Parkinson–White syndrome causes supraventricular tachycardia (SVT).

▶ Explain the need for referral to a paediatric cardiologist in order to decide on medium- to long-term management of the condition.

▶ There is a possibility of recurrence, but a low risk of future children being affected.

▶ There is no family history of this condition.

▶ Emphasise that with the current interventions, such as electro-ablation, this is now a curable condition with an excellent prognosis.

Your notes:

2: Breaking bad news

(e.g. please explain the results of ultrasound scan and its implications)

This is a 9-minute station consisting of spoken interaction. You will have up to 2 minutes before the start of the station to read this sheet and prepare yourself. You may make notes on the paper provided.

When the bell sounds you will be invited into the examination room. Please take this instruction sheet with you. The examiner will not ask questions during the 9 minutes, but will warn you when you have approximately 2 minutes left.

You are not required to examine a patient.

The encounter should be focused on the task: you will be penalised for asking irrelevant questions or providing superfluous information. You will be marked on your ability to communicate, not the speed with which you convey information. You may not have time to complete the communication.

Role: Paediatric specialist registrar.

Setting: Postnatal ward.

You are talking to: Mr and Mrs Firth, parents of 2-day-old Tony.

Background information: Tony was born at term after an uncomplicated pregnancy to a primi mother. His birth weight was 3.35 kg. Routine newborn examination by the SHO on day 2 revealed a cardiac murmur. Subsequent review (with echo scan) by the consultant confirmed small muscular VSD. The parents are upset about the diagnosis, and also about the fact that this was not picked up on the antenatal scans.

Task: Tony's father is asking to speak to someone. You are the registrar on call. The consultant has gone home. Explain to the parents the diagnosis and the planned management.

Points to consider:

▶ Explain the diagnosis of hole in the heart with pictures/diagrams, and allow time for the parents to take in this information.
▶ What are their main concerns?
▶ Do they know anyone in the family, or anyone else, with such a problem?
▶ Hole in the heart is the commonest heart problem in newborn babies, with an incidence of roughly 3 to 4 in 1000. Tony remains well in himself, and this small hole is unlikely to cause him any problems. His progress will be closely monitored in the specialist clinic. It is unlikely that he will require any treatment. There is every chance that the hole may close on its own in due course as a result of growth of muscle within the heart. In the event that it does not close spontaneously, it can be fixed surgically, with excellent outcome, but this is not something to consider at this stage.
▶ Antenatal scans, although very useful technology, have limitations and remain at best a screening tool. They would certainly *not* detect a small hole in the heart. This is why detailed clinical examination of all newborn babies must be carried out and further scans arranged as necessary.
▶ There will be an opportunity for Tony's parents to discuss specific issues with the specialist.
▶ Give the parents written information to take away with them.
▶ Explain that they will be able to take Tony home as planned and care for him like any other baby.
▶ Advise them to contact their GP if Tony has any difficulty at home with feeding, breathing, colour change, etc.
▶ Ascertain the parents' understanding.
▶ Ask them whether they have any other concerns.
▶ Finally, ask whether they have any further questions, and offer a repeat appointment if they still have unanswered questions or further concerns.

Your notes:

This is a 9-minute station consisting of spoken interaction. You will have up to 2 minutes before the start of the station to read this sheet and prepare yourself. You may make notes on the paper provided.

When the bell sounds you will be invited into the examination room. Please take this instruction sheet with you. The examiner will not ask questions during the 9 minutes, but will warn you when you have approximately 2 minutes left.

You are not required to examine a patient.

The encounter should be focused on the task: you will be penalised for asking irrelevant questions or providing superfluous information. You will be marked on your ability to communicate, not the speed with which you convey information. You may not have time to complete the communication.

Role: Neonatal registrar working in a busy tertiary-level unit.

Setting: Side room on the neonatal unit.

You are talking to: Mrs Lewis, mother of 2-week-old Bernard.

Background information: Bernard was born at 25 weeks' gestation, weighing 700 grams. He is now 2 weeks old and remains ventilator dependent. Clinical assessment and subsequent echo scan show a large patent ductus arteriosus (PDA). It has been planned to start Bernard on medical treatment with indomethacin.

Task: You need to explain to Mrs Lewis the treatment plan and the potential outcome following medical therapy.

Points to consider:

▶ PDA is common. Approximately 8 in every 1000 children have some form of congenital heart disease, and of these, around 15% have PDA.

▶ Almost all preterm babies born at 25 weeks' gestation, like Bernard, will have a patent duct.

▶ A patent duct is normal before the baby is born, and most close between 1 and 6 weeks of age.

▶ Draw a diagram. This makes it much easier to visualise and understand the diagnosis.

▶ Explain that normally the 'pink' blood and the 'blue' blood do not mix. However, the duct allows the two to mix.

▶ Without treatment, we are unlikely to make any progress in terms of reducing respiratory support (i.e. coming off the ventilator).

▶ This is because there is excess blood flow to the lungs, which makes them 'wet and stiff.'

▶ The treatment involves administering indomethacin. (Think of this medicine as similar to strong aspirin.)

▶ There is no guarantee that this medicine will work. The typical response rate is less than 50%.

▶ The side-effects of indomethacin include renal impairment (although this is always transient), reduced urine output, and weight gain.

▶ How will Bernard's progress be monitored? He will need a follow-up scan at the end of the treatment course to find out whether the duct has closed.

▶ For those babies who do not respond to treatment, the next step in management is surgical ligation, but this would be discussed with Mrs Lewis at a later date if it became necessary to do so.

▶ Confirm her understanding, and ask whether she has any questions. Offer to arrange for her to have a meeting with Bernard's consultant.

Your notes:

This is a 9-minute station consisting of spoken interaction. You will have up to 2 minutes before the start of the station to read this sheet and prepare yourself. You may make notes on the paper provided.

When the bell sounds you will be invited into the examination room. Please take this instruction sheet with you. The examiner will not ask questions during the 9 minutes, but will warn you when you have approximately 2 minutes left.

You are not required to examine a patient.

The encounter should be focused on the task: you will be penalised for asking irrelevant questions or providing superfluous information. You will be marked on your ability to communicate, not the speed with which you convey information. You may not have time to complete the communication.

Role: Neonatal registrar working in a busy tertiary-level unit.

Setting: Side room in the neonatal unit.

You are talking to: Mrs Smith, mother of Lillie.

Background information: Lillie was born at 24 weeks' gestation, weighing 620 grams. She is now 4 weeks old and remains ventilator dependent. Clinical assessment and subsequent echo scan showed a large patent duct. Lillie received a 6-day course of indomethacin. A repeat echo scan has shown the medical therapy to be ineffective. She still has a large duct. Your consultant has decided that Lillie will need transfer to the regional cardiac unit, where she will undergo duct ligation. Without surgical ligation Lillie will not be successfully weaned from the ventilator.

Task: Please explain the procedure of PDA ligation to Mrs Smith with a view to obtaining her consent to the procedure. Mrs Smith will have an opportunity to speak to the operating surgeons. However, consent should be obtained in case Mrs Smith is unable to accompany Lillie.

Points to consider:

▶ First you need to establish Mrs Smith's level of understanding of

PDA. Given that Lillie has already received a course of medical therapy, she may have some level of previous knowledge.

▶ Consider repeating a basic explanation of what a PDA is. Use a diagram here to aid visualisation of Lillie's problem.

▶ Again reinforce just how common PDA is in preterm babies, in order to offer some reassurance to Mrs Smith.

▶ What is her understanding of Lillie's current condition?

▶ You need to be quite clear that without surgical duct ligation it would be highly unlikely that Lillie would manage without respiratory support (the ventilator). The longer she remains on the breathing machine, the higher her risk of developing chronic lung disease will be.

▶ You then need to explain the actual procedure of duct ligation, including the potential complications.

▶ Mention that Mrs Smith would have the opportunity to speak to the operating surgeon at the tertiary centre. However, it is important that you are able to gain consent now in case she is unable to travel and accompany Lillie.

▶ Clarify her understanding, and offer her written information to take away with her.

▶ Provide a copy of the consent form, and check whether she has any further questions.

Your notes:

••

This is a 9-minute station consisting of spoken interaction. You will have up to 2 minutes before the start of the station to read this sheet and prepare yourself. You may make notes on the paper provided.

When the bell sounds you will be invited into the examination room. Please take this instruction sheet with you. The examiner will not ask questions during the 9 minutes, but will warn you when you have approximately 2 minutes left.

You are not required to examine a patient.

The encounter should be focused on the task: you will be penalised for asking irrelevant questions or providing superfluous information. You will be marked on your ability to communicate, not the speed with which you convey information. You may not have time to complete the communication.

••

Role: Paediatric specialist registrar.

Setting: Neonatal unit, tertiary level.

You are talking to: Mrs Blackburn, mother of 5-day-old Charlie.

Background information: Charlie was born at 26 weeks' gestation and had a birth weight of 670 g. He is now 5 days old, and remains stable on ventilatory support. He has had an ultrasound scan of the head. This shows grade 2 intraventricular haemorrhage on the right side. There are no parenchymal changes.

Task: Explain to Charlie's mother the results of the scan and its significance.

Points to consider:

▶ Explore Mrs Blackburn's understanding of the reasons for the head scan.
▶ State that this is similar to the scan that she had during pregnancy.
▶ This is something that is done routinely for premature babies. It can be done easily at the bedside without risk of radiation exposure, and can provide useful information about the structure of the brain, as well as evidence of bleeding within the water spaces (ventricles) and abnormalities in the white matter (bundle of nerve

fibres/wires). Emphasise that scans do not tell us anything about brain function.

▶ It is useful to draw a diagram to show the ventricles and surrounding parenchyma.

▶ The scan shows that Charlie has a blood clot within the water space on the right side. This does not require any treatment, and most such cases resolve over time. However, there is a possibility that it will get bigger, and we will be monitoring this through subsequent scans.

▶ Reassure her that there are no parenchymal changes (i.e. changes in the rest of the brain), although it may take a few weeks for these to show up.

▶ Explain that about 1 in 2 very premature babies may have neurodevelopmental problems later. This is why all such infants will require long-term follow-up.

▶ Whilst this risk exists for Charlie, the scan findings do not help to define the nature and extent of these difficulties.

▶ Offer to speak to Mrs Blackburn again if she has any other questions.

▶ Explain that she will have an opportunity to discuss the scan results with a consultant.

Your notes:

This is a 9-minute station consisting of spoken interaction. You will have up to 2 minutes before the start of the station to read this sheet and prepare yourself. You may make notes on the paper provided.

When the bell sounds you will be invited into the examination room. Please take this instruction sheet with you. The examiner will not ask questions during the 9 minutes, but will warn you when you have approximately 2 minutes left.

You are not required to examine a patient.

The encounter should be focused on the task: you will be penalised for asking irrelevant questions or providing superfluous information. You will be marked on your ability to communicate, not the speed with which you convey information. You may not have time to complete the communication.

Role: Neonatal registrar working in a busy DGH.

Setting: Outpatient clinic.

You are talking to: Mrs Briggs, mother of 4-month-old Thomas.

Background information: Thomas has been referred by his GP, who has heard a heart murmur during a routine examination. Thomas is an otherwise healthy baby, who was born at term. He is making excellent developmental progress and is thriving. There is no relevant family history.

Thomas has had an echo scan performed by your consultant, which reveals a small ventricular septal defect. This does not require treatment at present, and will probably close spontaneously.

Task: Please explain the diagnosis of ventricular septal defect to Mrs Briggs.

Points to consider:

▶ Start the consultation by asking how Thomas is. Does Mrs Briggs know why her GP has referred her here?

▶ Explain that Thomas has had a scan of his heart and you are going to explain what these pictures have shown.

▶ Thomas has a small *ventricular septal defect (VSD)*, which is a small hole in the heart.

▸ You need to reassure the mother at this point. The diagnosis sounds very alarming, so explain that you are going to draw her a diagram to explain exactly what this means.

▸ VSD is a type of congenital heart disease, which means that Thomas was born with it. It is common; about 4 in every 1000 babies have some form of heart defect.

▸ Now draw a very basic diagram showing the two atria, two ventricles and a small VSD. Explain, using simple terminology, about 'blue blood' and 'pink blood', and the fact that usually there is no mixing, but the small hole allows some mixing.

▸ Then consider using a structured approach:
  — presentation
  — investigations
  — management
  — prophylactic antibiotics
  — prognosis.

▸ Finally, having explained all of this, draw it together by summarising what this means for Thomas.

▸ Thomas is a healthy baby with a small VSD. Most VSDs of this size will close spontaneously. Mrs Briggs should continue to treat him as a normal baby.

▸ Acknowledge that this must come as a shock to her and that you have given her a lot of information. Provide reassurance and written information.

▸ Thomas will be seen here again for review. It may be possible to provide a contact telephone number for a cardiac liaison nurse so that if Mrs Briggs is worried or has further questions she will be able to contact the appropriate person.

Your notes:

This is a 9-minute station consisting of spoken interaction. You will have up to 2 minutes before the start of the station to read this sheet and prepare yourself. You may make notes on the paper provided.

When the bell sounds you will be invited into the examination room. Please take this instruction sheet with you. The examiner will not ask questions during the 9 minutes, but will warn you when you have approximately 2 minutes left.

You are not required to examine a patient.

The encounter should be focused on the task: you will be penalised for asking irrelevant questions or providing superfluous information. You will be marked on your ability to communicate, not the speed with which you convey information. You may not have time to complete the communication.

Role: Paediatric specialist registrar.

Setting: Postnatal ward.

You are talking to: Mrs Dowson, mother of 2-day-old Adam.

Background information: Adam was born at term after an uncomplicated pregnancy to a primip mother. His birth weight was 3.6 kg. Routine newborn examination by an SHO on day 2 revealed a cardiac murmur. You have since confirmed this finding yourself.

Task: Please inform Mrs Dowson of your finding/diagnosis and planned management.

Points to consider:

▶ Explain your findings and allow time for Mrs Dowson to take in this information.

▶ Does she know any other children/members of the family who have had a heart condition since birth?

▶ It is not uncommon to find a noise (murmur) when listening to a baby's heart. This can sometimes just be due to the way that blood flows around the heart, but in a small minority due to the abnormal structure of the heart. Emphasise that Adam is well in himself, breathing comfortably in room air, has normal pulses and oxygen levels in blood (oxygen saturation), and antenatal scans were reported to be normal. Hence it is less likely that Adam could have a serious underlying heart condition.

▶ Explain that you will be referring Adam to a specialist paediatrician, who will assess him either before discharge or in clinic within a week and be responsible for ongoing follow-up, if indicated.

▶ There will be an opportunity for Mrs Dowson to discuss specific issues with the specialist.

▶ Give her written information to take away with her.

▶ Explain that she will be able to take Adam home as planned and care for him like any other baby.

▶ Advise her to contact her GP if Adam has any problems at home with feeding, breathing, colour change, etc.

▶ Ascertain her understanding of what you have told her.

▶ Does she have any other concerns?

▶ Finally, ask whether she has any further questions, and offer a repeat appointment if she still has unanswered questions or further concerns.

Your notes:

This is a 9-minute station consisting of spoken interaction. You will have up to 2 minutes before the start of the station to read this sheet and prepare yourself. You may make notes on the paper provided.

When the bell sounds you will be invited into the examination room. Please take this instruction sheet with you. The examiner will not ask questions during the 9 minutes, but will warn you when you have approximately 2 minutes left.

You are not required to examine a patient.

The encounter should be focused on the task: you will be penalised for asking irrelevant questions or providing superfluous information. You will be marked on your ability to communicate, not the speed with which you convey information. You may not have time to complete the communication.

Role: Paediatric registrar working in a busy DGH.

Setting: Side room in children's outpatient clinic.

You are talking to: Hannah, aged 15 years, and her mother, Mrs Lowes.

Background information: Hannah has been attending the endocrine clinic over the last 4 weeks with a long history of weight loss, fine tremor and eye signs.

Task: Please explain the diagnosis of Graves' disease to Hannah and her mother.

Points to consider:

▶ First establish whether Hannah and her mother know why they have been asked to attend clinic today.
▶ Outline the basic structure of this consultation for them:
— Explain that the results of the tests that have been done show that Hannah has Graves' disease, which is the cause of her symptoms.
— Explain what Graves' disease is – an autoimmune disorder involving many systems in the body, including the thyroid gland, the eyes and sometimes the skin.

— Clinical symptoms: weight loss, fatigue, tremor, increased heart rate, appetite, inability to tolerate hot climates, palpitations, proximal myopathy, eye signs (chemosis, exophthalmos, lid lag, lid retraction, ophthalmoplegia).
— Underlying cause: autoimmune disorder caused by thyroid-stimulating immunoglobulins.
— Diagnosis: Made by blood tests, which usually show high levels of thyroxine with low TSH levels. (These will need to be explained – use a diagram to explain the basic physiology of the thyroid gland.) Antithyroid antibodies may also be present.
— Treatment: Divide into three main categories; medical, surgical and radio-iodine.
▶ Confirm their understanding of what you have told them, explain immediate management, provide written information and arrange follow-up.

Your notes:

This is a 9-minute station consisting of spoken interaction. You will have up to 2 minutes before the start of the station to read this sheet and prepare yourself. You may make notes on the paper provided.

When the bell sounds you will be invited into the examination room. Please take this instruction sheet with you. The examiner will not ask questions during the 9 minutes, but will warn you when you have approximately 2 minutes left.

You are not required to examine a patient.

The encounter should be focused on the task: you will be penalised for asking irrelevant questions or providing superfluous information. You will be marked on your ability to communicate, not the speed with which you convey information. You may not have time to complete the communication.

Role: Paediatric specialist registrar.

Setting: Postnatal ward.

You are talking to: Mrs Smith, mother of 2-day-old Toby.

Background information: Toby was born at term after an uncomplicated pregnancy to a primi mother. His birth weight was 3.8 kg. Routine newborn examination by an SHO on day 2 confirmed a dislocated hip on the left side.

Task: Please inform Mrs Smith of your finding/diagnosis and planned management.

Points to consider:

▶ Explain your diagnosis and allow time for Mrs Smith to take in this information.
▶ Ascertain her understanding of this condition.
▶ What are her main concerns?
▶ Does she know any other children who have had dislocated hip since birth?
▶ Explain that you will be referring Toby to an orthopaedic surgeon, who will be responsible for his ongoing management and follow-up.

- Early diagnosis is important, as in Toby's case, for a good outcome without surgical intervention.
- There will be an opportunity for Mrs Smith to discuss specific issues with the specialist.
- Most babies will improve with a splint (Pavlik's), and they tolerate this treatment very well without much pain or discomfort.
- Give Mrs Smith written information to take away with her.
- Finally, ask whether she has any further questions, and offer a repeat appointment if she still has unanswered questions or further concerns.

Your notes:

This is a 9-minute station consisting of spoken interaction. You will have up to 2 minutes before the start of the station to read this sheet and prepare yourself. You may make notes on the paper provided.

When the bell sounds you will be invited into the examination room. Please take this instruction sheet with you. The examiner will not ask questions during the 9 minutes, but will warn you when you have approximately 2 minutes left.

You are not required to examine a patient.

The encounter should be focused on the task: you will be penalised for asking irrelevant questions or providing superfluous information. You will be marked on your ability to communicate, not the speed with which you convey information. You may not have time to complete the communication.

Role: Neonatal registrar working in a busy DGH.

Setting: Side room on the postnatal ward.

You are talking to: Mrs Flanders, mother of baby Kate, who is 8 hours old.

Background information: Kate was born at term weighing 5.2 kg after an uneventful pregnancy. It had been a very difficult labour, and Kate was delivered by forceps. The midwife who is caring for Kate thinks she has Erb's palsy as a result of the difficult delivery, and has asked you to explain this to her mother, who is worried about the position of Kate's arm. She is an otherwise healthy baby.

Task: Please meet Mrs Flanders and explain the diagnosis of Erb's palsy and future management you feel is appropriate.

Points to consider:

▶ First congratulate Mrs Flanders on the birth of Kate, and acknowledge that you understand she had a very difficult delivery.
▶ Enquire after her health at this point. If she is in a great deal of pain she will be unable to concentrate on what you are saying.
▶ What are her concerns?
▶ Try to structure your conversation as follows:

— Kate has Erb's palsy – explain what this is.
— Explain why it has occurred.
— What is the underlying lesion?
— Management/treatment.
— Course and prognosis.
- Overall you can reassure her that this is not a permanent condition. It is in fact a common brachial plexus injury following difficult births.
- Physiotherapy will play an important role, and she will be taught some passive limb exercises.
- Make a follow-up appointment and refer Kate to a paediatric physiotherapist.
- Ensure that you have offered a full explanation which Mrs Flanders understands.
- Offer written information if appropriate.

Your notes:

This is a 9-minute station consisting of spoken interaction. You will have up to 2 minutes before the start of the station to read this sheet and prepare yourself. You may make notes on the paper provided.

When the bell sounds you will be invited into the examination room. Please take this instruction sheet with you. The examiner will not ask questions during the 9 minutes, but will warn you when you have approximately 2 minutes left.

You are not required to examine a patient.

The encounter should be focused on the task: you will be penalised for asking irrelevant questions or providing superfluous information. You will be marked on your ability to communicate, not the speed with which you convey information. You may not have time to complete the communication.

Role: Paediatric registrar working in a busy tertiary hospital.

Setting: Side room within children's outpatient department.

You are talking to: Mrs Wayper, mother of 6-month-old Jack.

Background information: Jack has an atrial septal defect (ASD). He has just attended follow-up clinic with your consultant. He is making excellent progress and is an otherwise healthy baby. Your consultant has asked you to talk to Mrs Wayper, as she remains unclear about what the diagnosis means and the future management of the condition.

Task: Please meet Mrs Wayper and explain the diagnosis of atrial septal defect and the likely future management.

Points to consider:

▶ Explain what you have been asked to discuss with her.
▶ What does she understand by the term *atrial septal defect* or *ASD*?
▶ Structure your conversation to make it easier for you both:
— Draw a diagram – this makes explanation much easier.
— Congenital heart disease is common, occurring in around 8 in 1000 babies, with approximately 10% having ASD, like Jack.
— Explain how babies usually present – with an asymptomatic murmur.

— What investigations they need: ECG, CXR, echocardiogram, possibly cardiac catheterisation.
— Management: usually 'umbrella' closure in the fourth or fifth year of life.
— Consequences of being left untreated.
— Prophylactic antibiotic use during surgery or dental work is no longer recommended (NICE Guideline).

▶ Offer written information and ensure her understanding.
▶ Jack will be followed up in clinic and if she has any further queries you would be happy to arrange another meeting.

Your notes:

This is a 9-minute station consisting of spoken interaction. You will have up to 2 minutes before the start of the station to read this sheet and prepare yourself. You may make notes on the paper provided.

When the bell sounds you will be invited into the examination room. Please take this instruction sheet with you. The examiner will not ask questions during the 9 minutes, but will warn you when you have approximately 2 minutes left.

You are not required to examine a patient.

The encounter should be focused on the task: you will be penalised for asking irrelevant questions or providing superfluous information. You will be marked on your ability to communicate, not the speed with which you convey information. You may not have time to complete the communication.

Role: A paediatric registrar working in the paediatric intensive-care unit within a busy DGH.

Setting: Relatives' room attached to the paediatric intensive-care unit.

You are talking to: Brian, the 20-year-old cousin of 4-year-old Dylan, who is currently being cared for in your unit.

Background information: Dylan has been on your unit for 48 hours following a road traffic accident. Earlier tests have confirmed brainstem death. His parents have asked you to wait until the relatives arrive before switching off the ventilator. They have asked you to explain the situation to Brian, who is very close to Dylan and is having difficulty understanding the situation.

Task: Please meet with Brian and explain why the ventilator is being switched off. Try to answer any questions he may have.

Points to consider:

▶ Express your sympathy about meeting in such sad and difficult circumstances.
▶ What is Brian's understanding of the situation at present?
▶ Explain that as a result of the accident, Dylan's brain has suffered

such massive injury that it is no longer able to function. This is known as 'brainstem death.'

▶ At the moment the machine or ventilator is doing all the work for Dylan, as his brain is no longer sending the signals which tell his body to breathe.

▶ Once the brain has been injured in this way it cannot recover. When we disconnect Dylan from the breathing machine he will stop breathing.

▶ Explain briefly that the brainstem test is carried out by two doctors, and it determines whether any parts of Dylan's brain are working.

▶ Dylan's test confirmed that this part of his brain has died. This means that there is no chance of survival or recovery.

▶ Dylan is not in pain and is not aware of his surroundings.

▶ His parents specifically requested that the ventilator should not be switched off until he got here, so that he would have the opportunity to say goodbye to Dylan.

▶ This is a very sad situation, and you are sorry for their terrible loss.

▶ Give Brian time to digest the information.

▶ Would he like some time alone? Or would he perhaps like you to take him to spend some time with Dylan and his family?

▶ This is a traumatic situation. There is help and support available both now and in the future if needed.

Your notes:

This is a 9-minute station consisting of spoken interaction. You will have up to 2 minutes before the start of the station to read this sheet and prepare yourself. You may make notes on the paper provided.

When the bell sounds you will be invited into the examination room. Please take this instruction sheet with you. The examiner will not ask questions during the 9 minutes, but will warn you when you have approximately 2 minutes left.

You are not required to examine a patient.

The encounter should be focused on the task: you will be penalised for asking irrelevant questions or providing superfluous information. You will be marked on your ability to communicate, not the speed with which you convey information. You may not have time to complete the communication.

Role: Paediatric registrar working in a busy DGH.

Setting: Room in children's outpatient department.

You are talking to: Mrs Christie Langford, mother of 10-day-old Alicia.

Background information: Alicia was born at term after an uncomplicated pregnancy. She has been at home since 2 days of age, and has been making good progress. She can sometimes be slow to feed, but is otherwise a healthy baby. There is no relevant family history. Alicia has a 3-year-old brother, Harry, who is fit and well.

Alicia's midwife rang Mrs Langford and asked her to attend an appointment in the outpatient department to discuss the results of her newborn screening test.

Task: A heel-prick blood sample was taken from Alicia when she was 5 days old. Following this she had a further venous sample taken. The results have shown that she has congenital hypothyroidism. Please inform Mrs Langford of this result and what the immediate management will be.

Points to consider:

▶ You need to start by asking whether Mrs Langford knows why she has been asked to attend today.

- Does she know what the newborn blood spot screening looks for?
- Then introduce the subject of congenital hypothyroidism.
- Give a simple explanation of the function of the thyroid gland.
- Congenital hypothyroidism is common, affecting 1 in 3500–4000 babies.
- It is usually a result of absent thyroid tissue.
- Untreated babies develop permanent physical and mental disability. However, there is an effective treatment.
- You will need to offer reassurance to Alicia's mother, who is likely to be very anxious.
- There is a simple and effective treatment – thyroxine – which when started early, as in Alicia's case, prevents intellectual deterioration and growth delay.
- Treatment will be started today, and Alicia will be seen and monitored regularly.
- Provide contact telephone numbers for support, and offer written information together with a follow-up appointment.
- It is important to let her midwife, health visitor and GP know about the diagnosis and treatment.
- Offer telephone contact in a day or two to provide support.

Your notes:

This is a 9-minute station consisting of spoken interaction. You will have up to 2 minutes before the start of the station to read this sheet and prepare yourself. You may make notes on the paper provided.

When the bell sounds you will be invited into the examination room. Please take this instruction sheet with you. The examiner will not ask questions during the 9 minutes, but will warn you when you have approximately 2 minutes left.

You are not required to examine a patient.

The encounter should be focused on the task: you will be penalised for asking irrelevant questions or providing superfluous information. You will be marked on your ability to communicate, not the speed with which you convey information. You may not have time to complete the communication.

Role: Neonatal specialist registrar working in a busy neonatal unit of a DGH.

Setting: Side room on the neonatal unit.

You are talking to: Mr Jackson, father of William, who is now 6 hours old.

Background information: William was born at 36 weeks' gestation via emergency Caesarean section for fetal distress and polyhydramnios. He was well at birth and did not require any resuscitation. After his first feed he went blue and became apnoeic. He was transferred to the neonatal unit. On passing a nasogastric tube, the tube curled in the oesophagus, which was confirmed on the chest X-ray. Air was also seen in the stomach. His mother is still unwell after the section, and is being cared for in the high-dependency unit. William's father is anxious to talk to you.

Task: Please talk to Mr Jackson about the likely diagnosis of tracheo-oesophageal fistula and the initial management of the condition.

Points to consider:

▶ Clarify Mr Jackson's understanding of the current situation.

▶ Consider using diagrams to explain the diagnosis.
▶ After each stage of explanation confirm his understanding. Acknowledge that this is a difficult time for him, and that there is a lot of information to take in at once.
▶ William's condition will require surgery and transfer to a paediatric surgical unit.
▶ Explain briefly what he should expect, but confirm that the surgeons will explain the procedure in detail when they arrive at the surgical unit. They can expect an excellent outcome following surgery.
▶ Explain that William may have a heart scan (echo scan) and blood test for chromosomes to rule out a few other conditions that may be associated with oesophageal atresia. Reassure him that clinical examination is not suggestive of any such associations.
▶ Assure him that he can come and see William on the neonatal unit prior to transfer, and that as soon as his wife is well enough she too can see her baby.
▶ Offer him written information and leaflets to aid your explanation.

Your notes:

This is a 9-minute station consisting of spoken interaction. You will have up to 2 minutes before the start of the station to read this sheet and prepare yourself. You may make notes on the paper provided.

When the bell sounds you will be invited into the examination room. Please take this instruction sheet with you. The examiner will not ask questions during the 9 minutes, but will warn you when you have approximately 2 minutes left.

You are not required to examine a patient.

The encounter should be focused on the task: you will be penalised for asking irrelevant questions or providing superfluous information. You will be marked on your ability to communicate, not the speed with which you convey information. You may not have time to complete the communication.

Role: Paediatric registrar.

Setting: Cubicle on the paediatric day unit.

You are talking to: Mrs Morrison, mother of 17-month-old Callum.

Background information: Callum is a previously fit and well 17-month-old boy. He was referred to the day unit by his general practitioner with a 5-day history of diarrhoea and vomiting. His GP was concerned about his level of hydration, and referred him to you for a second opinion. After taking a history and examining Callum, you feel that he is less than 5% dehydrated, and arrange to admit him to the children's ward for rehydration therapy. While examining Callum you note that he has peri-orbital and scrotal oedema. A urine dipstick reveals that he has 4+ of protein, consistent with a diagnosis of nephrotic syndrome. His blood pressure is 72 systolic.

Task: Please explain the diagnosis of nephrotic syndrome to Mrs Morrison.

Points to consider:

▶ First ask Mrs Morrison whether she has any ideas about what is causing Callum to be unwell.

▶ After examining Callum and doing an initial test on his urine, you can tell her that he has a condition called *nephrotic syndrome*.

▶ Has she heard of this or does she know anything about it?

▶ Explain that you appreciate that this has come as rather a shock to her, and you are going to take things slowly and explain what nephrotic syndrome is and also the initial management. She can interrupt and ask questions at any time, and if she does not understand something you have said, she should just ask and you will go over it again.

▶ In your own words, give a brief explanation of nephrotic syndrome. It is a disorder that affects the kidneys. Normally the kidneys work by tightly controlling what the body absorbs and getting rid of the waste material, excreting it as urine. In nephrotic syndrome the kidneys become 'leaky.' You could describe this as like having a bucket with holes in it, so that water and bigger particles can now pass through.

▶ One of the problems that this causes is letting protein through so that it is excreted in Callum's urine. We showed that he had protein in his urine by doing the dipstick test.

▶ We think of nephrotic syndrome as a disorder which has three main components:
  — proteinuria = protein in the urine (i.e. 'leaky' kidney)
  — hypoalbuminaemia = too little protein in the blood, caused by protein loss in the urine
  — oedema = swelling of the eyes and scrotum, and loss of fluid from the circulation.

▶ In childhood, if we look at the kidney cells under a microscope we see a change known as minimal change glomerulonephritis. This occurs in about 85% of cases.

▶ Nephrotic syndrome occurs in about 2 in 100 000 of the population.

▶ The mainstay of treatment is oral steroids, and most children will respond within 7 to 10 days. You will also do some further blood and urine tests.

▶ Depending on the time available, you can also mention complications, relapse and prognosis.

▶ This is a lot of information to take in at one sitting. Provide Mrs Morrison with written information, and then arrange a further meeting either later that day or the following day.

▶ Confirm that she has understood the information you have given her.

Your notes:

This is a 9-minute station consisting of spoken interaction. You will have up to 2 minutes before the start of the station to read this sheet and prepare yourself. You may make notes on the paper provided.

When the bell sounds you will be invited into the examination room. Please take this instruction sheet with you. The examiner will not ask questions during the 9 minutes, but will warn you when you have approximately 2 minutes left.

You are not required to examine a patient.

The encounter should be focused on the task: you will be penalised for asking irrelevant questions or providing superfluous information. You will be marked on your ability to communicate, not the speed with which you convey information. You may not have time to complete the communication.

Role: Paediatric specialist registrar working in a busy DGH.

You are talking to: Mrs Watson, mother of 5-year-old Joshua.

Setting: Side room on the paediatric ward.

Background information: Joshua is a previously fit and healthy little boy who has been admitted to your ward after having been unwell over the last 5–7 days. He has been diagnosed with Kawasaki disease and has been commenced on immunoglobulin and aspirin. His mother is aware of the diagnosis, but has asked to talk to you because she feels that she did not understand much of what was explained to her yesterday.

Task: Please explain the diagnosis, treatment and management of Kawasaki disease to Mrs Watson, and try to answer any questions she may have.

Points to consider:

▶ Start by finding out what Mrs Watson understands by the term *Kawasaki disease*.

▶ Invite her to interrupt and ask questions at any time.

▶ Consider breaking the information down into sub-headings as shown below. This will make it easier for you to structure your explanation, and also easier for Mrs Watson to follow what you are saying, using signposting.

— What Kawasaki disease is.
— General characteristics.
— What causes the disease.
— How the diagnosis is made.
— Investigations.
— Recommended treatment.
— Course and prognosis.
— Summary of the key points.

▶ Acknowledge that this is a lot of information to take in at one time. Offer her written information to take away with her, and also the opportunity to meet again to discuss any further questions she may have.

Your notes:

This is a 9-minute station consisting of spoken interaction. You will have up to 2 minutes before the start of the station to read this sheet and prepare yourself. You may make notes on the paper provided.

When the bell sounds you will be invited into the examination room. Please take this instruction sheet with you. The examiner will not ask questions during the 9 minutes, but will warn you when you have approximately 2 minutes left.

You are not required to examine a patient.

The encounter should be focused on the task: you will be penalised for asking irrelevant questions or providing superfluous information. You will be marked on your ability to communicate, not the speed with which you convey information. You may not have time to complete the communication.

Role: Paediatric registrar working in a busy DGH.

Setting: Paediatric outpatient clinic.

You are talking to: Mr and Mrs Johnson, parents of Chelsea, a 2-year-old girl.

Background information: Chelsea has been under your care since birth. She was adopted by Mr and Mrs Johnson at the age of 6 weeks, having been in foster care since birth. Her birth mother was a 15-year-old heroin addict who also had significant dependence on alcohol.

Chelsea has subtle facial dysmorphism and mild global developmental delay. Her parents have asked to discuss the diagnosis of fetal alcohol syndrome.

Task: Please explain to Mr and Mrs Johnson what is meant by the diagnosis of fetal alcohol syndrome.

Points to consider:

- Establish whether Mr and Mrs Johnson have any prior knowledge of the syndrome.
- There are no set diagnostic criteria.
- The syndrome consists of a collection of neurodevelopmental

and behavioural problems associated with alcohol intake during pregnancy.
- The exact amount of alcohol taken in pregnancy which is needed to cause the syndrome is not known.
- It is thought that even moderate amounts of alcohol consumed during pregnancy may reduce birth weight.
- Clinical features associated with fetal alcohol syndrome:
  - small for gestational age
  - postnatal – faltering growth (previously failure to thrive)
  - facial dysmorphism – saddle-shaped nose, maxillary hypoplasia, short palpebral fissures, epicanthic folds, absent philtrum
  - microcephaly.
- Other associations:
  - mild to moderate developmental delay, in particular speech and language delay, with poor spatial awareness
  - congenital heart disease
  - other system abnormalities – renal defects
  - skeletal deformities – affecting limbs, spine and digits.
- Confirm their understanding and try to give them an opportunity to ask further questions.
- Offer written information, a management plan and follow-up as appropriate.

Your notes:

This is a 9-minute station consisting of spoken interaction. You will have up to 2 minutes before the start of the station to read this sheet and prepare yourself. You may make notes on the paper provided.

When the bell sounds you will be invited into the examination room. Please take this instruction sheet with you. The examiner will not ask questions during the 9 minutes, but will warn you when you have approximately 2 minutes left.

You are not required to examine a patient.

The encounter should be focused on the task: you will be penalised for asking irrelevant questions or providing superfluous information. You will be marked on your ability to communicate, not the speed with which you convey information. You may not have time to complete the communication.

Role: Paediatric registrar working in a busy DGH.

Setting: Side room on the paediatric day unit.

You are talking to: Nikita, an 8-year-old girl, and her mother, Mrs Rahman.

Background information: Nikita is a previously fit and well child who has presented to your unit with a rash, mainly on her buttocks and lower limbs, and painful ankles. A diagnosis of Henoch–Schönlein purpura (HSP) has been made. As the registrar working on the unit that day, you have been asked to explain the diagnosis to Nikita's mother.

Task: Please explain the diagnosis of Henoch–Schönlein purpura (HSP) to Mrs Rahman.

Points to consider:

▶ Has Mrs Rahman heard of HSP before and does she know anything about it?

▶ Again there is a lot of information to cover and you only have 9 minutes. Consider using the following sub-headings to structure your conversation:
— What HSP is.
— Epidemiology.

— Underlying pathology.
— Diagnosis.
— Clinical features – go through each system that is affected in turn, in particular highlighting renal and joint involvement, as these are the two areas that cause parents and children most concern.
— Investigations.
— Treatment and management.
— Follow-up.
— Course and prognosis.

▶ Acknowledge that you have given Mrs Rahman a great deal of information, and reassure her that you do not expect her to retain it all.

▶ Offer her written information to take away with her, and ensure that she has understood what you have told her about management and follow-up.

▶ Arrange a set follow-up appointment, but also provide contact numbers for telephone support.

Your notes:

This is a 9-minute station consisting of spoken interaction. You will have up to 2 minutes before the start of the station to read this sheet and prepare yourself. You may make notes on the paper provided.

When the bell sounds you will be invited into the examination room. Please take this instruction sheet with you. The examiner will not ask questions during the 9 minutes, but will warn you when you have approximately 2 minutes left.

You are not required to examine a patient.

The encounter should be focused on the task: you will be penalised for asking irrelevant questions or providing superfluous information. You will be marked on your ability to communicate, not the speed with which you convey information. You may not have time to complete the communication.

Role: Paediatric registrar working in a busy DGH.

Setting: Clinic room in the children's outpatient department.

You are talking to: Mrs Smith, mother of 10-day-old Joshua.

Background information: Joshua was born at 38 weeks' gestation via emergency Caesarean section due to failure to progress and fetal distress. He was born in good condition and required no resuscitation. He was discharged home at 2 days of age bottle feeding well, and has continued to make good progress. Mrs Smith's midwife has been to see her and Joshua at home to inform them that there is a raised immunoreactive trypsin level on his Guthrie card test. The local hospital protocol states that Joshua will attend the outpatient clinic to discuss the result further. Joshua has two older siblings, both of whom are thriving and developmentally age appropriate. There is no family history of cystic fibrosis.

Task: Please discuss the Guthrie card test result with Mrs Smith, explain what the diagnosis means and discuss further management.

Points to consider:

▶ Ask Mrs Smith if she knows why she has been asked to attend the hospital today.

119

▶ Confirm her understanding of the Guthrie card test (metabolic conditions, PKU, congenital hypothyroidism, immunoreactive trypsin or IRT).

▶ Explain that IRT is used as a screening tool for cystic fibrosis.

▶ Explain what we mean by the word 'screening test', i.e. those babies who have a positive result on their screening blood test have an increased risk of having the disease in question, in this case cystic fibrosis. However, it does not confirm that Joshua definitely has the disease.

▶ Check her knowledge of cystic fibrosis.

▶ Provide a basic explanation – problem with the sweat glands, resulting in the production of thick, sticky secretions. Too much salt in the sweat. This can affect many systems in the body, leading to poor weight gain, recurrent chest infections and gut problems.

▶ It is a life-limiting condition. However, with current treatment children can have a good quality of life. You can briefly mention treatment if you feel this is appropriate. The main point would be the multi-disciplinary team, and highlighting of antibiotic use and physiotherapy.

▶ You need to emphasise that at this stage we do not have a definite diagnosis.

▶ Confirming the diagnosis – gold standard is the sweat test, and genetic testing looking for the abnormal gene (more than 78% of cases in the UK have deltaF508).

▶ You may also need to touch upon the subject of Joshua's siblings, who would also need to have a sweat test arranged.

▶ Acknowledge that this information must have come as a shock to Mrs Smith, and that it is a very difficult situation for her.

▶ Arrange a further appointment to confirm/refute the diagnosis, and offer her leaflets to read with contact telephone numbers.

▶ Check her understanding of what you have told her, and clarify any outstanding issues.

Your notes:

This is a 9-minute station consisting of spoken interaction. You will have up to 2 minutes before the start of the station to read this sheet and prepare yourself. You may make notes on the paper provided.

When the bell sounds you will be invited into the examination room. Please take this instruction sheet with you. The examiner will not ask questions during the 9 minutes, but will warn you when you have approximately 2 minutes left.

You are not required to examine a patient.

The encounter should be focused on the task: you will be penalised for asking irrelevant questions or providing superfluous information. You will be marked on your ability to communicate, not the speed with which you convey information. You may not have time to complete the communication.

Role: You are a paediatric specialist registrar working in a DGH.

Setting: Outpatient clinic room.

You are talking to: Mr and Mrs Smith, parents of 7-week-old Bethany.

Background information: During a routine check, Bethany's GP heard a continuous heart murmur and has referred her to the paediatric department for a cardiology opinion. She was born at term, has been gaining weight well and has no other medical problems. Her development is age appropriate.

> Task: Your consultant has performed an echo scan which shows a small patent ductus arteriosus (PDA). Bethany's heart is otherwise functioning well. Your consultant has asked you to explain the diagnosis to her parents.

Points to consider:

▶ First establish the parents' understanding of why they have been referred today.

▶ PDA is common; approximately 8 in every 1000 children have some form of congenital heart disease, of whom around 15% have PDA.

▶ PDA is normal before the baby is born, and in most cases it closes between 1 and 6 weeks of age.

▶ It is very common in preterm infants.

▶ Draw a diagram, as this makes it much easier to visualise and understand the diagnosis.

▶ Explain that normally the 'pink blood' and the 'blue blood' do not mix. However, the duct allows the two to mix.

▶ There are different options for management (i.e. medical and surgical ligation). However, in this case the duct is tiny and Bethany's heart is working well.

▶ You will confirm management with your consultant, but at the present time Bethany does not need any treatment and you will monitor her progress in clinic.

▶ Summarise, and offer Bethany's parents a diagram and written information.

▶ Ask them whether they have any other questions.

Your notes:

This is a 9-minute station consisting of spoken interaction. You will have up to 2 minutes before the start of the station to read this sheet and prepare yourself. You may make notes on the paper provided.

When the bell sounds you will be invited into the examination room. Please take this instruction sheet with you. The examiner will not ask questions during the 9 minutes, but will warn you when you have approximately 2 minutes left.

You are not required to examine a patient.

The encounter should be focused on the task: you will be penalised for asking irrelevant questions or providing superfluous information. You will be marked on your ability to communicate, not the speed with which you convey information. You may not have time to complete the communication.

Role: Neonatal registrar in a quiet DGH.

Setting: Side room of postnatal ward.

You are talking to: Mrs Janine Tall, mother of Billie, now 12 hours old.

Background information: Janine Tall, a 42-year-old librarian, delivered her third child at home. She was then transferred to the postnatal ward for a check-up. Janine and her midwife have noticed that Billie does not look like her other children, and have therefore asked for a paediatrician to assess the baby.

Your SHO has seen Billie and reports that there are clear features of Down syndrome.

Task: Please break the news to Mrs Tall that you believe that Billie has Down syndrome.

Points to consider:

▶ Offer your congratulations on the birth of Billie.
▶ Does Mrs Tall know why you have been asked to see her?
▶ Does she have a partner, friend or relative whom she would like to be present? (Make sure that a nurse or midwife, preferably one who knows the mother, is present.)

- Ask Mrs Tall whether there were any concerns during pregnancy. Did she have any form of antenatal screening?
- Be honest and open, and state that you feel it is very likely that Billie has Down syndrome, which will need to be confirmed by a blood test.
- Ask whether she has heard of Down syndrome or knows any children with Down syndrome.
- Explain the diagnosis, trisomy 21 (i.e. three copies instead of two of chromosome number 21), the most common cause of severe learning difficulty.
- It is common, occurring in 1 in 1000 live births.
- There is a lot of information you could give her, but for now offer a small amount and acknowledge that this is a difficult time for her.
- Explain briefly the clinical features, associated problems (heart, thyroid and eyes) and the need for multi-disciplinary team involvement.
- Emphasise that children with this condition, particularly those without a heart abnormality, do well without requiring much medical input. As far as you know, Billie does not have a heart problem.
- Immediate management is to encourage bonding. Discuss breastfeeding.
- Summarise and check Mrs Tall's understanding of what you have told her, and arrange a second meeting when you can give her further information.
- Provide her with written information and contact details, including telephone support numbers and relevant websites.

Your notes:

This is a 9-minute station consisting of spoken interaction. You will have up to 2 minutes before the start of the station to read this sheet and prepare yourself. You may make notes on the paper provided.

When the bell sounds you will be invited into the examination room. Please take this instruction sheet with you. The examiner will not ask questions during the 9 minutes, but will warn you when you have approximately 2 minutes left.

You are not required to examine a patient.

The encounter should be focused on the task: you will be penalised for asking irrelevant questions or providing superfluous information. You will be marked on your ability to communicate, not the speed with which you convey information. You may not have time to complete the communication.

Role: You are a specialist registrar working in the neonatal unit of a large DGH.

Setting: Relatives' room on the neonatal unit.

You are talking to: Mr and Mrs Parry, parents of Sarah, born 24 hours ago.

Background information: Sarah was born at 25 weeks' gestation by spontaneous vaginal delivery. She was extensively bruised at birth. Her ventilation settings have remained stable. At 8 hours of age Sarah was noted to be having frequent seizures which, although initially difficult to manage, are now well controlled on medication. Your consultant has performed a cranial USS which showed bilateral grade 3 intraventricular haemorrhage.

Task: Your consultant has asked you to explain the diagnosis of intraventricular haemorrhage to Sarah's parents, and to try to answer any questions they may have. He will join you in a short while to clarify any queries.

Points to consider:

▶ Explain that you are one of the doctors who have been caring for Sarah on the unit. Try to arrange to have a nurse present who has previously met the parents.

- Acknowledge that this is a difficult time for them, and ask how they are managing.
- What do they know about Sarah's current treatment?
- Go back to basics, and explain that Sarah was born very early, which can cause lots of problems. At the moment the ventilator is doing the work of Sarah's lungs, but she is coping well with this.
- Explain the seizures, which are due to abnormal electrical activity in her brain.
- A USS (jelly scan) was done to look for a possible cause of these fits. It has shown that Sarah has had a bleed within the water spaces (ventricles) inside her brain.
- The blood vessels in her brain are very delicate and can bleed very easily.
- Probably the biggest risk factor for this is being born very early, as Sarah was.
- You can explain the timing of bleeds and the Papile classification of periventricular–intraventricular haemorrhage (i.e. grades 1–4) if this will aid their understanding.
- There is no treatment indicated to 'control' bleeding, which will take a natural course.
- Sarah will have regular (twice weekly) monitoring of head size, as well as a head scan to assess the size of the ventricles to rule out the development of hydrocephalus (excess water inside brain).
- What does the future hold for them as a family? Always answer honestly, and if you do not know, say so, but offer to try to find out further information for them.
- Possible sequelae to think about – these include hydrocephalus and cerebral palsy.
- It is important to distinguish between a scan picture (which shows the structure of the brain) and how this relates to function. Brain scans do not inform us about brain function.
- Although there is a risk of neurodevelopmental delay, it is difficult to define the nature and severity of this. It will require long-term monitoring.
- At present Sarah is stable, but she has a long path ahead. You will keep them fully updated and can arrange regular contact. Ask if they have any questions, and check their understanding of what you have told them.

Your notes:

This is a 9-minute station consisting of spoken interaction. You will have up to 2 minutes before the start of the station to read this sheet and prepare yourself. You may make notes on the paper provided.

When the bell sounds you will be invited into the examination room. Please take this instruction sheet with you. The examiner will not ask questions during the 9 minutes, but will warn you when you have approximately 2 minutes left.

You are not required to examine a patient.

The encounter should be focused on the task: you will be penalised for asking irrelevant questions or providing superfluous information. You will be marked on your ability to communicate, not the speed with which you convey information. You may not have time to complete the communication.

Role: Neonatal specialist registrar working in a quiet DGH.

Setting: Side room on the postnatal ward.

You are talking to: Mrs Flanders, mother of Dylan, who is 8 hours old.

Background information: Dylan is the third child of Mrs Flanders. He was born at full term via normal delivery after an uneventful pregnancy. He did not require any resuscitation at birth, and has taken two bottle feeds well. His midwife, during a routine check of his oxygen saturation, found his saturation in air to be 84%. He was transferred to the neonatal unit and an echo scan has confirmed pulmonary stenosis. Your consultant is arranging transfer to the nearest cardiac centre.

Task: Please talk to Dylan's mother and explain the diagnosis to her.

Points to consider:

▶ First offer your congratulations on the birth of Dylan.
▶ Would she like a partner, friend or relative to be with her?
▶ Does she know why the midwife asked you to review Dylan?
▶ Explain that there are many reasons why a baby can have low oxygen saturations. In Dylan's case we have done a scan of his heart which has shown us why his saturations are lower than normal.

▶ Begin to explain the diagnosis of pulmonary stenosis. Acknowledge that this will be a difficult time for her, and reassure her that you can go over things until she understands what you are telling her.

▶ Draw a simple diagram showing the atria, ventricles, narrowed pulmonary artery and the patent duct.

▶ Pulmonary stenosis is a form of congenital heart disease, which means that he was born with it. It is common, occurring in about 8 in 1000 babies, of whom around 10% have the same problem as Dylan.

▶ The important thing now is to give Dylan a medicine (into a vein) which keeps the duct open. Use your diagram to show her how this is done.

▶ You are arranging transfer to a tertiary centre where he will undergo further assessment. He may have either a surgical procedure or balloon dilatation.

▶ They will explain his management in detail when he arrives.

▶ Summarise, and allow ample opportunity for discussion and further questions.

Your notes:

··

This is a 6-minute station. You will have 3 minutes beforehand to read this sheet and prepare yourself. You may take the sheet with you into the station, but you must return it at the end.

··

Role: An ST3 GP trainee.

Setting: GP surgery.

You are talking to: Agatha, the mother of 8-year-old Maxine.

Background information: Agatha has noticed recently that Maxine looks pale, and she has been complaining of abdominal pain occasionally. She has been noted to have rather pale stools that are difficult to flush. She underwent an emergency appendicectomy 6 months ago. She has a normal appetite and is growing appropriately for her age. She is doing well at school.

Maxine's mother has recently been diagnosed with coeliac disease after suffering from 'irritable bowel syndrome' for many years. She has had two endoscopies, which were very traumatic for her. She is worried that her daughter may have to go through the same traumatic experience during the investigations to diagnose coeliac disease.

The family are all vegetarians.

Examination reveals that Maxine is pale. Her abdomen is normal on examination.

Task: To discuss the investigations to diagnose coeliac disease, and to address the anxieties that Maxine's mother has about the tests.

YOU ARE NOT EXPECTED TO GATHER THE REST OF THE MEDICAL HISTORY DURING THIS CONSULTATION.

Points to consider:

▶ Explore the mother's ideas and specific concerns. She is clearly worried that Maxine may have coeliac disease. She may not want her to undergo painful procedures such as biopsy. She may want to know whether Maxine will grow normally, and also whether Ben (Maxine's 4-year-old brother) could develop this condition in the future.

▶ Reassure the mother and adopt an empathetic attitude.
▶ Explain the steps involved in the diagnosis of coeliac disease.
▶ Reassure the mother that endoscopy and biopsy would be performed under general anaesthetic.
▶ Explain the inheritance of the condition and the risk of Maxine's brother developing it.
▶ Explain the use of the screening test for Maxine's brother if he does not have any symptoms.
▶ It is likely that iron-deficiency anaemia is linked to coeliac disease, and this will require iron supplementation.
▶ Mention the need for liaison with the school nurse.
▶ Offer some literature in the form of information leaflets to the mother.

Your notes:

3: Consent

(e.g. please explain why you need to do a lumbar puncture, with a view to obtaining consent)

This is a 9-minute station consisting of spoken interaction. You will have up to 2 minutes before the start of the station to read this sheet and prepare yourself. You may make notes on the paper provided.

When the bell sounds you will be invited into the examination room. Please take this instruction sheet with you. The examiner will not ask questions during the 9 minutes, but will warn you when you have approximately 2 minutes left.

You are not required to examine a patient.

The encounter should be focused on the task: you will be penalised for asking irrelevant questions or providing superfluous information. You will be marked on your ability to communicate, not the speed with which you convey information. You may not have time to complete the communication.

Role: Paediatric specialist registrar.

Setting: Side room on a paediatric ward.

You are talking to: Helen Crowther, mother of 4-year-old Alexander.

Background information: Alexander is being treated with IV antibiotics for a clinical diagnosis of meningitis. When he first presented he had signs of altered conscious level, and was too unwell to undergo a lumbar puncture. He spent 24 hours on the PICU, and is now stable enough to be transferred to the ward. He has had a normal CT scan, and the decision was made on the morning ward round to do a lumbar puncture that morning. *Helen is against the idea of Alexander having a lumbar puncture.*

Task: Explain to Helen why it is important to perform an lumbar puncture, and answer any questions she may have.

Points to consider:

▶ Ask Helen what she has been told about Alexander's condition and treatment so far.

▶ Explain that you would like to do a lumbar puncture, which involves using a special needle to obtain a small sample of fluid from the spine. This is the fluid which travels up the spine and surrounds the brain.

▶ It is important to isolate the organism, as this will not only confirm whether you are using the right antibiotics, but it will also determine the length of treatment needed.

▶ Explain the procedure, including the use of local anaesthetic, sedation and the position adopted.

▶ She may respond by pointing out that you are already giving him the treatment for meningitis, so why can you not carry on without doing a lumbar puncture. Reiterate the need for isolation of the organism (appropriate choice of antibiotics based on sensitivity) and guide to length of treatment. It is also important from a public health perspective.

▶ Be prepared to discuss the possible complications and contraindications if she asks about them.

▶ Some centres obtain written consent.

▶ Confirm Helen's understanding of what you have told her.

Your notes:

This is a 9-minute station consisting of spoken interaction. You will have up to 2 minutes before the start of the station to read this sheet and prepare yourself. You may make notes on the paper provided.

When the bell sounds you will be invited into the examination room. Please take this instruction sheet with you. The examiner will not ask questions during the 9 minutes, but will warn you when you have approximately 2 minutes left.

You are not required to examine a patient.

The encounter should be focused on the task: you will be penalised for asking irrelevant questions or providing superfluous information. You will be marked on your ability to communicate, not the speed with which you convey information. You may not have time to complete the communication.

Role: Paediatric specialist registrar.

Setting: Relatives' room in A&E department.

You are talking to: Justine Maple, 18-year-old mother of 4-month-old Leah.

Background information: Leah was born pre-term at 28 weeks' gestation. She had a stormy neonatal course, and was ventilated for 3 weeks. She was discharged home 2 weeks ago on 0.6 l of nasal cannula oxygen, and was due for follow-up with the neonatal team in 2 days. Her parents found Leah in bed with them in the early hours of the morning and realised that she was not breathing. Paramedics had tried to resuscitate her, but she was pronounced dead on arrival at A&E. A probable diagnosis of sudden infant death syndrome has been made and explained to her parents.

Task: Ask Justine for consent to perform a muscle biopsy on Leah.

Points to consider:

▶ Express your sympathy for the tragic circumstances in which you are meeting Justine.

▶ Ask whether she would like her partner, or a friend, relative or nurse to be present with her.

- Gently ask her if she is able to give consent for you to perform a muscle biopsy on Leah.
- Explain why you want to do this – to try to exclude some inherited/ metabolic diseases which may have caused Leah's death.
- Highlight the importance of this for future pregnancies. Be sensitive, as many parents in such circumstances feel that they do not want another child, although many later change their minds.
- Briefly explain the procedure, and again be sensitive to Justine's needs, giving only as much information as she is able to deal with, sufficient for informed consent.
- The results can take many weeks and sometimes months, but the parents will not have to wait all this time for the body to be released so that they can make funeral arrangements.
- Is there anything that you have not made clear and that Justine wishes to discuss?

Your notes:

This is a 9-minute station consisting of spoken interaction. You will have up to 2 minutes before the start of the station to read this sheet and prepare yourself. You may make notes on the paper provided.

When the bell sounds you will be invited into the examination room. Please take this instruction sheet with you. The examiner will not ask questions during the 9 minutes, but will warn you when you have approximately 2 minutes left.

You are not required to examine a patient.

The encounter should be focused on the task: you will be penalised for asking irrelevant questions or providing superfluous information. You will be marked on your ability to communicate, not the speed with which you convey information. You may not have time to complete the communication.

Role: You are a paediatric specialist registrar working on the day unit of a busy DGH.

Setting: Cubicle on the day unit.

You are talking to: Mr and Mrs Lucas, parents of 15-week-old Ethan.

Background information: Ethan was born at term by normal delivery, weighing 6 lb 4oz. Over the last 2 weeks he has had increasing episodes of vomiting, and has seen his GP on numerous occasions because the health visitor was worried about poor weight gain. After your assessment, a capillary blood gas analysis shows a picture of metabolic alkalosis, and a USS confirms the diagnosis of pyloric stenosis. After speaking to the paediatric surgeons at the receiving tertiary centre, you are planning to transfer Ethan for surgery. He is haemodynamically stable.

Task: Please inform Mr and Mrs Lucas of the diagnosis of pyloric stenosis and the expected management, with a view to obtaining consent.

Points to consider:

▶ Explain the diagnosis using a diagram, as it is much easier to visualise the food pipe, stomach and pyloric opening this way.

▶ Explain 'pyloric stenosis' in non-medical terms. It is a narrowing of the part of the stomach that connects to the small intestine. Due to this narrowing it makes it harder for the milk to pass through, and therefore Ethan vomits.

▶ Be careful when using the term 'pyloric tumour.' Think about the parents' interpretation of the word 'tumour.'

▶ Explain that the condition is common, more so in firstborn males, and that there may be a family history.

▶ You can briefly explain the operation if you understand it (i.e. Ramstedt's pyloromyotomy). Otherwise say that you are not going into detail as the surgical team will explain this before the consent is taken.

▶ Reassure the parents appropriately. Although there are risks with any surgery, the prognosis is excellent. Most babies feed within 24 hours of surgery and tolerate the procedure well, rapidly regaining their lost weight postoperatively.

▶ Confirm their understanding, and give them your diagram or written information sheet.

Your notes:

....

This is a 6-minute station. You will have 3 minutes beforehand to read this sheet and prepare yourself. You may take the sheet with you into the station, but you must return it at the end.

....

Role: A GP.

Setting: A GP surgery.

You are talking to: Mrs Rashi, the mother of 2-week-old baby Rajiv.

Background information: Mr and Mrs Rashi have recently immigrated to the UK from India where the prevalence of tuberculosis is high. Their firstborn child, Rajiv, was born at the local hospital, which has a policy that requires a return to the clinic for a BCG vaccine if necessary. The couple have been informed by the health visitor about the need for a BCG immunisation. The parents seem very unwilling for their son to be immunised with BCG.

Other information: The family lives in an area populated by other immigrant families from different parts of the world. Mrs Rashi's mother died of a chest condition, but she is not sure of its exact nature.

Task: To advise Mrs Rashi about the need for BCG immunisation.

Points to consider:

▷ Try to explore the mother's concern about BCG vaccine. It is possible that she is alarmed by the idea of her son having an injection this early in life, or she may know someone who had delayed wound healing after receiving the vaccine. She may just want her son to have the same routine injections as other infants. She may be worried about the potential complications of immunisation. Understanding her specific concerns will allow you to address these more effectively.

▷ Explain the need for BCG immunisation for infants who come from high endemic areas.

▷ Discuss the risk of acquiring tuberculous infection as a result of contact with relatives who have travelled from other endemic areas, or with local immigrant families in the neighbourhood.

▶ Reassure the mother that BCG immunisation will take time to heal and leaves a small scar, but this is necessary to indicate that immunisation has been successful.

▶ BCG vaccine offers good protection against severe forms of tuberculosis (such as TB meningitis and disseminated TB).

▶ Earlier vaccination gives better protection. You could consider giving BCG with 'routine' vaccines at 2 months, but it would be better for the baby to be protected as soon as possible, given the potential risks of exposure.

Your notes:

4: Critical incidents

(e.g. please talk to this parent whose child has been given the wrong drug)

••

This is a 9-minute station consisting of spoken interaction. You will have up to 2 minutes before the start of the station to read this sheet and prepare yourself. You may make notes on the paper provided.

When the bell sounds you will be invited into the examination room. Please take this instruction sheet with you. The examiner will not ask questions during the 9 minutes, but will warn you when you have approximately 2 minutes left.

You are not required to examine a patient.

The encounter should be focused on the task: you will be penalised for asking irrelevant questions or providing superfluous information. You will be marked on your ability to communicate, not the speed with which you convey information. You may not have time to complete the communication.

••

Role: You are a paediatric specialist registrar working in a busy DGH.

Setting: Doctor's office on the paediatric ward.

You are talking to: Dr Matthew Hamilton, a colleague.

Background information: Matthew is a fourth-year specialist registrar who has recently returned to clinical work after taking two years out to perform some research. There have been concerns from nursing staff and other medical staff that he is under-performing at work, and on a number of occasions you have smelt alcohol on his breath while at work. The nursing sister on the ward has also been concerned that

Matthew has been drinking while on night shift, and has asked you to speak to him.

Task: Please talk to Matthew, broach the subject of an alcohol problem and discuss any further concerns he may have.

Points to consider:

▶ This is a difficult conversation to have with a colleague. Be honest and say that you find this uncomfortable but you need to talk to him about how he is managing returning to clinical work after a long period away.
▶ Ask him how he thinks he is coping.
▶ Is there anything in particular that he is finding difficult? Is there any help or support you can offer him?
▶ If he does not volunteer the information, again be honest and say that there have been some general concerns about his health, in particular worries related to drinking both at home and at work.
▶ Is this a problem he is aware of?
▶ He may either acknowledge the problem or deny it.
▶ Explain that there are serious concerns as he could potentially be putting patients at risk, and he will need to seek professional guidance.
▶ This is a disciplinary offence of which the General Medical Council needs to be informed. Liaise with senior consultants.
▶ Offer to help him to find support, either from professional organisations, the occupational health service or his GP. It would be important to talk to his consultant or educational supervisor. Again, offer him support in doing this.
▶ Finally, reassure him that you want to help him. He may wish to meet with you again, either at work or for support outside work.
▶ Be aware that he may refuse to acknowledge the problem, and may become angry or aggressive. You need to stay very calm, but reiterate how serious this is and that you would need to talk to your consultant if he felt unable to do so.

Your notes:

This is a 9-minute station consisting of spoken interaction. You will have up to 2 minutes before the start of the station to read this sheet and prepare yourself. You may make notes on the paper provided.

When the bell sounds you will be invited into the examination room. Please take this instruction sheet with you. The examiner will not ask questions during the 9 minutes, but will warn you when you have approximately 2 minutes left.

You are not required to examine a patient.

The encounter should be focused on the task: you will be penalised for asking irrelevant questions or providing superfluous information. You will be marked on your ability to communicate, not the speed with which you convey information. You may not have time to complete the communication.

Role: Paediatric specialist registrar.

Setting: Side room on the paediatric surgical ward.

You are talking to: Mrs Barr, mother of 5-year-old Jack.

Background information: Jack has epilepsy which has been fully investigated. He has had a normal MRI scan, and on medication he is normally well controlled. He is otherwise growing and developing normally. He was admitted to the paediatric surgical ward the previous day for tonsillectomy. He was initially first on the list, which had been pre-arranged so that he would be nil by mouth for as short a time as possible, allowing him to continue with his anti-epileptic medication.

Due to an emergency, his operation was delayed until late in the afternoon. Jack has now returned to the ward and has managed a drink.

Your paediatric surgical colleague has asked you to speak to his mother, as she has become angry and upset that Jack has suffered due to the delay.

Task: Speak to Mrs Barr and explore her concerns.

Points to consider:

▶ Explain to Mrs Barr that you have been asked to speak to her from a paediatric point of view.

- Tell her that you understand that this situation has been difficult for her and you are sorry she is upset.
- Let her explain her worries and concerns, responding where appropriate.
- Highlight the fact that perhaps it was lack of communication that led to her becoming upset.
- Explain that emergencies cannot be predicted, and sometimes elective surgery does get delayed because of these.
- Focus on the fact that Jack does not seem to have suffered, the operation went well, without complications, and he is now on the ward and tolerating an oral diet.
- Offer to speak with the surgical team on her behalf and see where things can be improved so that other children and parents are not put in the same position in future.
- If she would like to take the matter further, you can arrange for a meeting between herself and the consultant involved.
- Also offer her details of the Patient Advice and Liaison Service (PALS).
- You can fill in an incident form which highlights difficulties like these, so that if possible similar situations can be avoided in the future.
- Finally, you can offer to review Jack, especially if his mother is concerned about seizure control because he missed doses of anti-epileptics.
- Explain that you can be contacted again if she has any other concerns.

Your notes:

This is a 9-minute station consisting of spoken interaction. You will have up to 2 minutes before the start of the station to read this sheet and prepare yourself. You may make notes on the paper provided.

When the bell sounds you will be invited into the examination room. Please take this instruction sheet with you. The examiner will not ask questions during the 9 minutes, but will warn you when you have approximately 2 minutes left.

You are not required to examine a patient.

The encounter should be focused on the task: you will be penalised for asking irrelevant questions or providing superfluous information. You will be marked on your ability to communicate, not the speed with which you convey information. You may not have time to complete the communication.

Role: Paediatric registrar in a DGH.

Setting: Side room in the paediatric day unit.

You are talking to: Miss Bartley, mother of 2-year-old Jessica.

Background information: Jessica has attended the paediatric day unit with a 3- to 4-day history of coryzal symptoms and wheeze. She has been seen by your SHO, who has made a diagnosis of viral-induced wheeze. On admission Jessica was pyrexial and was given a dose of paracetamol. As the registrar you are asked to review her. When you look at the drug Kardex you query the dose of paracetamol. It transpires that the weight recorded by the admitting nurse was incorrect, as the scales had been set to pounds instead of kilograms. The dose of paracetamol was then worked out at 15 mg/kg, but on a working weight in pounds instead of kilograms.

Task: You need to talk to Jessica's mother and explain that there has been a drug error, how it occurred, and what your management will be now.

Points to consider:

▶ First introduce yourself and make sure that a nurse, preferably one who has been involved in Jessica's care, is present.

- Ask Miss Bartley if she would like her partner or a friend or relative to be with her during the discussion.
- You need to be honest and open and explain exactly what the drug error is and how it occurred.
- Reasure her that Jessica is very unlikely to come to any harm because of the increased dose.
- Explain what the management will involve. In 4 hours' time you will check the paracetamol level in Jessica's blood. Again emphasise that you expect it to be normal.
- You can then go on to explain the formal procedure of filling in incident forms, and informing senior nursing staff and the consultant responsible for Jessica.
- The aim is to assess the risk and to try to minimise any future risk to other children.
- This incident is being taken very seriously, and apologise to her that this has happened.
- She can put her concerns in writing if she feels that this is more appropriate.
- Reiterate the fact that she does not need to take this any further if she does not wish to, as you can ensure that you will be taking all of the relevant steps to try to prevent this from happening again.
- Concentrate on Jessica being well. You have realised the mistake and will work with the department to minimise future risk.
- Offer her the contact details of the Patient Advice and Liaison Service (PALS).
- You can also invite her to meet with the consultant and senior nursing staff if she would like the opportunity to discuss this further.

Your notes:

147

This is a 9-minute station consisting of spoken interaction. You will have up to 2 minutes before the start of the station to read this sheet and prepare yourself. You may make notes on the paper provided.

When the bell sounds you will be invited into the examination room. Please take this instruction sheet with you. The examiner will not ask questions during the 9 minutes, but will warn you when you have approximately 2 minutes left.

You are not required to examine a patient.

The encounter should be focused on the task: you will be penalised for asking irrelevant questions or providing superfluous information. You will be marked on your ability to communicate, not the speed with which you convey information. You may not have time to complete the communication.

Role: Registrar in a tertiary-level neonatal unit.

Setting: Side room in the neonatal unit.

You are talking to: Miss Cleaver, mother of 3-day-old Thomas.

Background information: Thomas was born pre-term at 26 weeks' gestation. He is otherwise stable on a ventilator for RDS. He has had a blood transfusion for anaemia (Hb 10). The blood bank technician has contacted you, stating that Thomas has been transfused with the wrong blood (rhesus positive instead of rhesus negative), due to an error. You have since assessed Thomas, who remains well and stable. You have also discussed this matter with the consultant haematologist and the neonatal consultant.

Task: You need to talk to Miss Cleaver and explain that there has been an error in blood transfusion, how it occurred and what your management will be now.

Points to consider:

▶ First introduce yourself and make sure that a nurse is present, preferably one who has been involved in Thomas's care.

▶ Ask Miss Cleaver if she would like her partner or a friend or relative to be with her during the discussion.

- You need to be honest and open and explain exactly what the error is and how it occurred.
- The incident is being taken very seriously, and apologise to her that this has happened.
- Reassure her that you have assessed Thomas and he remains stable. Preterm infants do not mount 'transfusion reaction.' There is no immediate intervention indicated according to expert advice from the haematology consultant.
- This incident may have implications for the future, as Thomas's immune system is sensitised and may produce antibodies. This situation will be monitored.
- You can then go on to explain the formal procedure of filling in critical incident forms, and informing senior nursing staff and the consultant responsible for Thomas.
- The aim is to assess the risk and to try to minimise any future risk to other children.
- She can put her concerns in writing if she feels that this is more appropriate.
- Offer her the contact details of the Patient Advice and Liaison Service (PALS).
- Reiterate the fact that she does not need to take this any further if she does not wish to, as you can ensure that you will be taking all of the relevant steps to try to prevent this from happening again.
- Concentrate on Thomas being well. A mistake has occurred and this will be dealt with in order to minimise future risk.
- Invite her to meet with the consultant and the unit manager if she would like the opportunity to discuss the matter further.

Your notes:

This is a 9-minute station consisting of spoken interaction. You will have up to 2 minutes before the start of the station to read this sheet and prepare yourself. You may make notes on the paper provided.

When the bell sounds you will be invited into the examination room. Please take this instruction sheet with you. The examiner will not ask questions during the 9 minutes, but will warn you when you have approximately 2 minutes left.

You are not required to examine a patient.

The encounter should be focused on the task: you will be penalised for asking irrelevant questions or providing superfluous information. You will be marked on your ability to communicate, not the speed with which you convey information. You may not have time to complete the communication.

Role: Neonatal specialist registrar working in a busy neonatal unit of a DGH.

Setting: Side room on the neonatal unit.

You are talking to: Mr Williamson, father of 3-day-old Jack.

Background information: Jack was born prematurely at 30 weeks' gestation. He is otherwise well and stable, and does not require any respiratory support or supplemental oxygen. It is planned for him to have intravenous antibiotics (penicillin and gentamicin) for 7 days because of group B streptococcus infection. You have been informed that he received the second gentamicin dose at 24 hours instead of 36-hourly as prescribed, due to an error.

> Task: Please talk to Mr Williamson and explain that there has been an error in giving the antibiotic, how it occurred, and what your management will be now.

Points to consider:

▶ Introduce yourself and make sure that a nurse is present.
▶ You need to be honest and open and explain exactly what the error is and how it occurred.
▶ Assure Mr Williamson that the incident is being taken very

seriously, and apologise to him that it has happened.

▶ Reassure him that Jack remains well and stable. He has not come to any harm as a result of having his antibiotic dose 12 hours earlier. His gentamicin level will be checked before he is given the next dose. Your plan is still to complete the full course of treatment as planned. Hearing screening will be arranged for Jack before discharge.

▶ You can then go on to explain the formal procedure of filling in incident forms, and informing senior nursing staff and the consultant responsible for Jack.

▶ Explain that the aim is to assess the risk and try to minimise any future risk to other children.

▶ Mr Williamson can put his concerns in writing if he feels this is more appropriate.

▶ Offer him the contact details of the Patient Advice and Liaison Service (PALS).

▶ Reiterate the fact that he does not need to take it any further if he does not wish to, as you can ensure that you will be taking all of the relevant steps to try to prevent this from happening again.

▶ Invite him to meet with the consultant and the unit manager if he would like the opportunity to discuss the matter further.

Your notes:

This is a 9-minute station consisting of spoken interaction. You will have up to 2 minutes before the start of the station to read this sheet and prepare yourself. You may make notes on the paper provided.

When the bell sounds you will be invited into the examination room. Please take this instruction sheet with you. The examiner will not ask questions during the 9 minutes, but will warn you when you have approximately 2 minutes left.

You are not required to examine a patient.

The encounter should be focused on the task: you will be penalised for asking irrelevant questions or providing superfluous information. You will be marked on your ability to communicate, not the speed with which you convey information. You may not have time to complete the communication.

Role: A paediatric specialty registrar (ST4) working in a district general hospital.

You are talking to: Chelsea, the adoptive mother of 4-year-old Trisha.

Setting: Children's outpatient clinic.

Background information: Trisha was seen in the day unit 5 weeks ago for constipation. She was prescribed Movicol and a review was arranged. Before you review the progress of Trisha's constipation, her mother asks you for the result of the urine test for Sanfilippo syndrome. There is no record in Trisha's notes of the test being ordered, but there is a result of a urine mucopolysaccharide assay which is clearly labelled as Trisha's, and which is normal.

The notes from the earlier review are signed by a junior colleague who has recently passed his MRCPCH Part 1. He had apparently told the mother that Trisha's coarse facial features were indicative of Sanfilippo syndrome, and that the urine test would confirm the diagnosis. He had ascertained that there was a family history of this condition in a natural cousin.

Task: To discuss the possible misdiagnosis with Trisha's adoptive mother.

YOU ARE NOT EXPECTED TO GATHER THE REST OF THE MEDICAL HISTORY DURING THIS CONSULTATION.

Points to consider:

▶ Establish the mother's understanding of the situation.

▶ Adopt a sensitive and sympathetic attitude to the mother's feelings.

▶ Encourage the mother to express her views.

▶ Understand the mother's anger and anxiety.

▶ Apologise for the distress caused to the mother.

▶ Avoid criticising or blaming your junior colleague.

▶ Negotiate whether a further assessment of Trisha by a clinical geneticist would be helpful now that the possibility has been raised.

▶ Demonstrate a basic knowledge of the presentation, diagnosis and prognosis of the mucopolysaccharidoses.

▶ Remember that a negative urine mucopolysaccharide screen does not completely exclude Sanfilippo syndrome.

▶ Refer the patient to a clinical geneticist rather than ordering specialised tests inappropriately.

Your notes:

5: Ethics

(e.g. please discuss the problem that Anna has refused to have any blood tests)

This is a 9-minute station consisting of spoken interaction. You will have up to 2 minutes before the start of the station to read this sheet and prepare yourself. You may make notes on the paper provided.

When the bell sounds you will be invited into the examination room. Please take this instruction sheet with you. The examiner will not ask questions during the 9 minutes, but will warn you when you have approximately 2 minutes left.

You are not required to examine a patient.

The encounter should be focused on the task: you will be penalised for asking irrelevant questions or providing superfluous information. You will be marked on your ability to communicate, not the speed with which you convey information. You may not have time to complete the communication.

Role: Neonatal specialist registrar.

Setting: Delivery room of the obstetric unit of a DGH.

You are talking to: Mr and Mrs Kirkbride.

Background information: Mrs Kirkbride has been admitted to the labour ward with ruptured membranes and preterm onset of labour at 26 weeks' gestation. She and her husband are concerned about the poor survival rate and high risk of disabilities among such survivors, and therefore *do not* want the neonatal team to resuscitate their new-born baby at delivery.

They have a 3-year-old daughter, Mia, who is in perfect health.

Mrs Kirkbride has received a course of steroid (betamethasone) since admission.

> Task: Explain to Mr and Mrs Kirkbride the proposed management plan options at delivery, and the rationale for this.

Points to consider:
- Explore the parents' understanding so far, and ask them whether they have had any opportunity to discuss the situation with the midwife and/or obstetrician.
- Have they had any experience (among family or friends) of extreme preterm babies?
- National (UK) data would suggest that about two out of three such babies will be expected to survive with modern treatment, and well over half of these are 'intact' without significant neurodevelopment issues by 2½ years of age. Babies who are born to mothers who have received steroid treatment have a better outcome. All such babies will need some help with breathing, usually either a mask or a tube in the windpipe.
- It would be reasonable to offer this level of help and support as part of 'early stabilisation' and *not* 'resuscitation.'
- If there is a good response to the above intervention (in terms of improved heart rate, colour and breathing), the baby will be admitted to the neonatal unit for ongoing care.
- However, if there is no response, it would not be appropriate to intervene with medications such as adrenaline and cardiac massage.
- The neonatal team will be present at the time of delivery to assess the condition of the baby at birth and the response to early intervention.
- Ask whether they have any other questions.
- Offer to come back and speak to them again if they have any other queries.
- They will have an opportunity to discuss any issues with the consultant on the neonatal unit.

Your notes:

This is a 9-minute station consisting of spoken interaction. You will have up to 2 minutes before the start of the station to read this sheet and prepare yourself. You may make notes on the paper provided.

When the bell sounds you will be invited into the examination room. Please take this instruction sheet with you. The examiner will not ask questions during the 9 minutes, but will warn you when you have approximately 2 minutes left.

You are not required to examine a patient.

The encounter should be focused on the task: you will be penalised for asking irrelevant questions or providing superfluous information. You will be marked on your ability to communicate, not the speed with which you convey information. You may not have time to complete the communication.

Role: Paediatric registrar working in a busy DGH.

Setting: Relatives' room on the paediatric ward.

You are talking to: Jenna, aged 15 years, and her parents, Mr and Mrs Jordan.

Background information: Jenna has been suffering from anorexia nervosa for the last 18 months. She has been an inpatient at the local adolescent eating disorders unit for 12 weeks. She was admitted to the acute medical ward as there were increasing concerns about her physical health. She is hypotensive and bradycardic. Jenna is co-operating to some extent and will eat low-calorie foods and sugar-free juices. However, she is refusing to stay on the unit, and is threatening to abscond.

On the advice of the consultant psychiatrist, as Jenna's parents agree to her being an inpatient, from a legal standpoint they are able to override Jenna's wishes. Another alternative would be to section Jenna. However, this is not felt to be necessary at present.

Task: Please talk to Jenna and her parents and explain that Jenna will remain an inpatient with her parents' consent.

Points to consider:

- First acknowledge that this is a very difficult situation for all involved.
- Explain what you have been asked to discuss with them (i.e. that Jenna will remain as an inpatient on your unit, certainly for the time being).
- Direct much of the conversation towards Jenna, irrespective of how difficult or uncommunicative she may be.
- Ask open questions – does Jenna know why she was transferred to this unit?
- You need to explain to Jenna that the opinion of both the medical staff caring for her and her parents is that the best place for her is as an inpatient on this unit. You can explain the reasons behind this (i.e. her poor physical health).
- At some point the issue of consent will most probably be raised. Legally Jenna cannot refuse treatment as she is 15 years old. Her parents have both given consent for her to be an inpatient, and this overrides her refusal.
- Another question that may be raised concerns sectioning Jenna under the Mental Health Act. Although this is an option, it is not necessary, because Jenna's parents are giving their consent.
- This will undoubtedly be a difficult conversation. Acknowledge this, and remain calm and in control.
- Always remember to be aware of your own limitations. You can arrange a meeting with your consultant and the psychiatric consultant involved in Jenna's care.

Your notes:

159

This is a 9-minute station consisting of spoken interaction. You will have up to 2 minutes before the start of the station to read this sheet and prepare yourself. You may make notes on the paper provided.

When the bell sounds you will be invited into the examination room. Please take this instruction sheet with you. The examiner will not ask questions during the 9 minutes, but will warn you when you have approximately 2 minutes left.

You are not required to examine a patient.

The encounter should be focused on the task: you will be penalised for asking irrelevant questions or providing superfluous information. You will be marked on your ability to communicate, not the speed with which you convey information. You may not have time to complete the communication.

Role: Paediatric registrar working in a busy DGH.

Setting: Adolescent bay of the children's ward.

You are talking to: Elaine, a 14-year-old girl who has been admitted following a paracetamol overdose.

Background information: Elaine is a previously fit and well 14-year-old girl. She was admitted via A&E following a paracetamol overdose. This was precipitated following an argument with her boyfriend and her best friend at school. Blood paracetamol levels confirm that she needs to be treated with Parvolex. Your SHO has asked you to speak to Elaine, as she is refusing all treatment. Her parents have been contacted and are on their way to the unit.

Task: Please talk to Elaine, and discuss the need for treatment and the likely outcome if she refuses treatment.

Points to consider:

 ▶ Ask Elaine whether she understands why you have been asked to come and speak to her.
 ▶ It will be important here to be firm but at the same time to build a rapport and gain her trust.
 ▶ Explore the reasons behind her taking the overdose:

- Home circumstances.
- School – academic progress, bullying, friendships.
- Peer pressure – smoking, alcohol, recreational drug use.
- Boyfriends and sexual relationships.

▶ Explore the details surrounding the actual overdose:
  - Was it planned or done on the spur of the moment?
  - What did she think would happen or want to happen when she took the tablets?
  - Did she tell anyone?
  - Did she write a suicide note?
  - Did she consume any alcohol?

▶ Explain that the blood tests show that there is a dangerous level of paracetamol in her body which could seriously affect her health. In particular it could damage her liver.

▶ This situation can, if left untreated, be life-threatening.

▶ Reassure her that you want to help her. It is very important that this treatment is started quickly in order to try to minimise any damage to her liver.

▶ Is she frightened of something in particular? For example, does she have a needle phobia, or is she worried about getting into trouble once her parents find out?

▶ She may eventually give you consent for treatment. However, if she refuses, you must be quite clear that legally she cannot refuse treatment at her age.

▶ You would need to involve senior consultants and her parents, and seek guidance from the Trust solicitor, the General Medical Council, the Medical Protection Society and colleagues in adolescent psychiatry.

Your notes:

This is a 9-minute station consisting of spoken interaction. You will have up to 2 minutes before the start of the station to read this sheet and prepare yourself. You may make notes on the paper provided.

When the bell sounds you will be invited into the examination room. Please take this instruction sheet with you. The examiner will not ask questions during the 9 minutes, but will warn you when you have approximately 2 minutes left.

You are not required to examine a patient.

The encounter should be focused on the task: you will be penalised for asking irrelevant questions or providing superfluous information. You will be marked on your ability to communicate, not the speed with which you convey information. You may not have time to complete the communication.

Role: A paediatric registrar working in a busy tertiary hospital.

Setting: Relatives' room on the paediatric ward.

You are talking to: Mr and Mrs Barncroft, parents of 11-year-old Joey.

Background information: Joey has severe Crohn's disease. He is now under the care of the paediatric surgeons, who feel that he needs a laparotomy with possible bowel resection. Joey and his parents are devout Jehovah's witnesses. The surgical team have asked if you will speak to them about possible blood transfusion before they come and take consent for the procedure.

> Task: Please meet with Mr and Mrs Barncroft and raise the possibility of blood transfusion both during the operation and post-operatively.

Points to consider:

▶ Introduce yourself and explain truthfully why you have been asked to come and talk to them.

▶ You may start off by saying something like 'I understand you may have very strong feelings about the use of blood products – how would you feel if it became necessary for Joey to receive a blood transfusion?'

- Reiterate that Joey would not routinely be given a transfusion. However, as in any operation, there is a risk of bleeding.
- If Joey was to lose a lot of blood during surgery, not giving him a transfusion might put his life at serious risk.
- This may be a very difficult and heated discussion, but regardless of your personal beliefs you must maintain control of the situation.
- Gauge the parents' reaction. It may be necessary to seek legal advice, involve the Trust solicitor, or contact the Medical Protection Society or the General Medical Council for further advice.
- There is the possibility of using a 'cell saver', but there will be a timescale factor to consider here.
- Allow the parents some time alone to take in what you have said. Involve senior medical staff and arrange a further meeting.
- Try to empathise and show that you appreciate that this must be a very difficult situation for them.

Your notes:

This is a 9-minute station consisting of spoken interaction. You will have up to 2 minutes before the start of the station to read this sheet and prepare yourself. You may make notes on the paper provided.

When the bell sounds you will be invited into the examination room. Please take this instruction sheet with you. The examiner will not ask questions during the 9 minutes, but will warn you when you have approximately 2 minutes left.

You are not required to examine a patient.

The encounter should be focused on the task: you will be penalised for asking irrelevant questions or providing superfluous information. You will be marked on your ability to communicate, not the speed with which you convey information. You may not have time to complete the communication.

Role: Neonatal registrar working in a busy tertiary referral centre.

Setting: Relatives' room on the neonatal unit.

You are talking to: Mr Wallace, a 33-year-old brick layer and father of Caleb, now 1 week old.

Background information: Caleb was born 1 week ago at 24 weeks' gestation weighing 650 grams. He was in poor condition at birth and has had a stormy course since then. He is difficult to ventilate, requiring high pressures and increasing amounts of oxygen. He has bilateral pneumothoraces that require chest drains. He is not being fed. At present he still requires two inotropes to maintain his perfusion. Despite this, he remains hypotensive and poorly perfused. He has not passed any urine for over 2 days, and has developed acute renal failure. Over the last 48 hours he has been fitting continuously despite being given increasing doses of anti-epileptics. Following an acute deterioration today, a repeat cranial ultrasound scan was performed which has revealed bilateral grade 4 intraventricular haemorrhages. The team involved in Caleb's care all agree that the appropriate action would be to withdraw care.

Mrs Wallace remains in the adult intensive-care unit following a complicated delivery.

Task: Discuss with Mr Wallace Caleb's current condition and the possible withdrawal of care.

Points to consider:

▶ Offer your condolences for meeting in such difficult circumstances.
▶ Does he wish a relative or friend to be with him to provide support?
▶ Enquire about the health of his wife.
▶ Explain that you are going to talk to him about Caleb.
▶ Find out what his understanding is of the current situation.
▶ Caleb is seriously unwell. Break down the information into systems (brain, lungs, heart, kidneys, gut) and go through each in turn. This will give more structure to the conversation and will also be easier for him to follow.
▶ At each stage stop and check his understanding. Ask whether there are any areas that he wishes you to go over.
▶ So far, none of the treatments that Caleb has received have had any positive effect. His deterioration has been relentless. There is no hope for him, and continuing intensive care indefinitely may just be prolonging his suffering.
▶ Introduce the concept of withdrawing care. Think about how you are going to explain this to him. Caleb is critically unwell, despite all of the medical treatment you are giving him, and his body is no longer able to fight.
▶ Explain the manner in which care would be withdrawn. The parents can be present if they wish, they can hold and cuddle Caleb, and he would be kept comfortable.
▶ Offer the opportunity for a religious service if appropriate.
▶ Discuss the support that will be available after Caleb has died.
▶ Arrange further meetings, and offer to go with Mr Wallace to see Caleb on the unit.

Your notes:

Role: Paediatric registrar working on the teenage oncology unit.

Setting: Relatives' room on the unit.

You are talking to: Mr and Mrs Bubb, parents of 14-year-old Jason.

Background information: Jason is currently an inpatient on your unit. He was referred from the local DHG with non-specific symptoms of malaise, pallor and cough. Following investigations, a diagnosis of leukaemia has been made. Both Jason and his parents are fully aware of the diagnosis and the treatment available.

Jason had previously been a fit and very active child, and played football competitively at regional level. His grandfather died 6 months ago from lung cancer, despite intensive treatment. Since he has been on the unit Jason has remained adamant about refusing all treatment.

Task: Jason's parents are very anxious, as despite lengthy discussions with Jason, he is refusing all treatment. Please discuss this issue with Jason's parents, as they wish to know their options.

Points to consider:

▶ Ask Jason's parents if they are aware of any particular issues which are worrying Jason and therefore leading to his refusal of treatment.

- Possible areas of concern include fear related to the death of his grandfather, anxiety, pain, and the side-effects of treatment.
- Do they believe that he is aware of the serious consequences of remaining untreated (i.e. death)?
- Who has talked to Jason so far? Has anyone talked with him on a one-to-one basis?
- Has he built a rapport with any of the doctors or nurses on the unit?
- At this point you can bring up the concept of 'Gillick competence' (now known as 'Fraser competence').
- It would be likely that if Jason continued to refuse treatment, permission to go ahead would be sought from court.
- This would be a last resort. The biggest risk is of alienating Jason completely from his parents and the medical staff. It would be preferable to resolve this issue without resorting to legal measures.
- Involve other agents in speaking to Jason (e.g. counsellor, psychologist), who are specially trained in talking with young people.
- Acknowledge his parents' anxiety, and the fact that this is a very difficult situation. You also need to understand how difficult this is for Jason and continue to offer support.
- Perhaps allowing Jason to meet with other young people on the unit may offer him some support and reassurance.
- Clarify a way forward (i.e. arrange a further meeting, possibly with a psychologist).
- Reassure Jason's parents that they are not alone, and that they are not the only parents who are faced with this situation. The multi-disciplinary team will support them as a family.

Your notes:

168

This is a 9-minute station consisting of spoken interaction. You will have up to 2 minutes before the start of the station to read this sheet and prepare yourself. You may make notes on the paper provided.

When the bell sounds you will be invited into the examination room. Please take this instruction sheet with you. The examiner will not ask questions during the 9 minutes, but will warn you when you have approximately 2 minutes left.

You are not required to examine a patient.

The encounter should be focused on the task: you will be penalised for asking irrelevant questions or providing superfluous information. You will be marked on your ability to communicate, not the speed with which you convey information. You may not have time to complete the communication.

Role: You are a paediatric registrar working in a large DGH with a 4-bedded intensive-care unit.

Setting: Relatives' room attached to the intensive-care unit.

You are talking to: Mr and Mrs Waller, parents of 3-year-old Demi.

Background information: Demi was involved in a road traffic accident 3 days ago and is currently a patient in intensive care. Despite intensive treatment, two consultants have confirmed that she is brain dead. Her parents have been kept fully updated and aware of the situation. They are waiting for relatives to arrive before switching off the life support machine.

You have been involved in Demi's care and have a good rapport with her parents.

Task: Please speak to Demi's parents and raise the issue of organ donation. (You are not expected to know the details of the actual process of organ donation.)

Points to consider:

‣ Express your condolences about meeting in such tragic circumstances.
‣ Be honest with them. Acknowledge that you need to talk to them

about a very sensitive issue which they may find difficult to discuss.

▶ You would like to raise the issue of organ donation.

▶ Pause here and let them take in what you have said.

▶ At this point you need to gauge the reaction of Demi's parents.

▶ Ask them if they have had any thoughts either now or previously regarding organ donation.

▶ Is it something they wish to discuss further?

▶ Emphasise that this is a very personal decision, and that no pressure will be put on them, whatever they decide.

▶ Briefly, if appropriate, offer some basic information. Over 3000 transplants are performed each year in the UK, the most common ones being kidney, heart, liver and cornea.

▶ Some parents find it comforting to think that something positive has come from such tragic circumstances.

▶ You need to be empathic and respond to the parents.

▶ Offer to arrange a meeting with the transplant co-ordinator.

▶ Give the parents an opportunity to ask questions, and acknowledge that this is a difficult time for them.

▶ Offer further support and a second meeting if organ donation is something they would like to consider.

Your notes:

This is a 9-minute station consisting of spoken interaction. You will have up to 2 minutes before the start of the station to read this sheet and prepare yourself. You may make notes on the paper provided.

When the bell sounds you will be invited into the examination room. Please take this instruction sheet with you. The examiner will not ask questions during the 9 minutes, but will warn you when you have approximately 2 minutes left.

You are not required to examine a patient.

The encounter should be focused on the task: you will be penalised for asking irrelevant questions or providing superfluous information. You will be marked on your ability to communicate, not the speed with which you convey information. You may not have time to complete the communication.

Role: Paediatric registrar working in a busy DGH.

Setting: Side room on the paediatric ward.

You are talking to: Emma Winter, a 14-year-old girl who is currently an inpatient on your ward.

Background information: Emma has been an inpatient for the last 4 days, following an appendicectomy. She is otherwise fit and well, with no known medical problems. You have just finished the ward round, during which you said that she could be discharged. Emma has asked to speak to you alone before she goes home, as she wants you to prescribe the oral contraceptive pill for her.

Task: Please arrange to meet with Emma and discuss the prescribing of the oral contraceptive pill, exploring any concerns that she may have.

Points to consider:

▶ First you need to clarify that Emma wants the OCP for contraception rather than for regulating her menstrual cycle.
▶ Enquire about the relationship she is in:
  — age of partner
  — whether it is her first sexual relationship

— whether she is using any contraception at present.

▶ Has she discussed the matter with her mother, aunt, older cousin, school nurse or GP? She needs to be encouraged to do so.

▶ Raise the subject of sexually transmitted infections. The OCP does not protect her from these. Discuss screening, the use of condoms, etc.

▶ Remind her she is under age, and that in the UK it is illegal to have sexual intercourse under the age of 16 years.

▶ Praise her for acting responsibly in seeking contraceptive advice.

▶ Discuss teenage pregnancies.

▶ Gillick/Fraser competence – legally you can prescribe the OCP if you consider her to be competent.

▶ It is important for her to see her GP. Again reassure her that this would remain confidential, but highlight the importance of follow-up, blood pressure monitoring, repeat prescriptions, smear tests and STI screening.

▶ If she would prefer not to attend a GP surgery, there are drop-in clinics held specifically for young people who need contraception. Encourage her partner to attend with her.

▶ You can arrange an appointment for her. Again reiterate how important it would be to talk to either her mother or another adult whom she trusts.

▶ Are there any other issues that she wishes to discuss?

▶ Arrange a meeting if appropriate, or provide contact details for the young people's clinic or GP surgery.

Your notes:

....

This is a 9-minute station consisting of spoken interaction. You will have up to 2 minutes before the start of the station to read this sheet and prepare yourself. You may make notes on the paper provided.

When the bell sounds you will be invited into the examination room. Please take this instruction sheet with you. The examiner will not ask questions during the 9 minutes, but will warn you when you have approximately 2 minutes left.

You are not required to examine a patient.

The encounter should be focused on the task: you will be penalised for asking irrelevant questions or providing superfluous information. You will be marked on your ability to communicate, not the speed with which you convey information. You may not have time to complete the communication.

....

Role: Neonatal registrar working in a tertiary-level neonatal unit.

Setting: Side room attached to the neonatal unit.

You are talking to: Helena Carter, a final-year medical student.

Background information: Helena is attached to the unit for a 6-week placement towards her student select module. She has attended a business ward round with your team. She was there when you approached the parents of Baby Edwards (27 weeks' gestation, day 3, currently ventilated for RDS and planned for extubation to nasal CPAP), for recruitment in an ongoing CPAP trial. Helena is uncomfortable about the idea of conducting research on newborn babies and children, and she wants to discuss this with you.

Task: Explain to Helena why it is ethical to conduct research studies on newborn babies, and answer any questions that she may have.

Points to consider:

▪ Make sure that you hold this discussion in a separate room where you are less likely to be disturbed.

▪ Try to understand what specific questions/concerns Helena has.

▪ The purpose of clinical research is to achieve an improved outcome for the patient population. If this is so, there is no reason whatsoever why newborn babies should not benefit from well designed and conducted studies. This is the only way we can move further forward in terms of providing medical care.

▶ In fact, neonatal intensive care, as a relatively new specialty, is a good example of vastly improved survival in preterm infants as a result of research – for example, the use of antenatal steroids, and surfactant treatment for RDS. This is further helped by improved perinatal care and use of modern technology.

▶ It is absolutely essential that any research is conducted within the research governance framework and that it meets the approval of ethics and research committees.

▶ There are safeguards put in place to ensure that studies are conducted properly.

▶ You could mention how the process of obtaining consent (i.e. from parents or guardian) is different.

▶ The parents are under no obligation to participate in the study. Their newborn baby will receive the same level of care whether they decide to participate or not. They are free to change their mind at any stage without having to give any explanation.

▶ Summarise what you have told Helena. You could briefly describe the ongoing unit studies.

▶ Ask her whether her concerns have been addressed.

Your notes:

Role: A GP registrar.

Setting: GP surgery.

You are talking to: Tarn, a 15-year-old girl, friend of Susan.

Background information: Tarn has come to see you with the excuse of bad period pains. In fact she is extremely concerned about her friend, Susan, who is also 15 years old. Over the last few months Susan has lost a lot of weight and has become very thin. She only eats salad, she skips lunch, and she exercises for about 4 hours each day. She regularly goes to the toilet after eating. Tarn has heard her being sick. Yesterday she found two bottles of laxatives in Susan's bedroom.

Task: To discuss Tarn's concerns about Susan.

YOU ARE NOT EXPECTED TO GATHER THE REST OF THE MEDICAL HISTORY DURING THIS CONSULTATION.

Points to consider:
▶ Listen sensitively to Tarn and understand her concerns.
▶ Susan needs to come and see her doctor and agree to disclosure.
▶ It would be unethical to speak to Susan's parents without obtaining her consent.
▶ Do not offer to discuss the matter with Tarn's parents.
▶ Emphasise that it would be unethical to discuss Susan's condition without her consent.
▶ Enquire further whether there are any underlying issues with regard to Tarn's health.
▶ There is no need to discuss anorexia in detail, but be prepared to discuss its management briefly with Tarn.

Your notes:

This is a 9-minute station consisting of spoken interaction. You will have up to 2 minutes before the start of the station to read this sheet and prepare yourself. You may make notes on the paper provided.

When the bell sounds you will be invited into the examination room. Please take this instruction sheet with you. The examiner will not ask questions during the 9 minutes, but will warn you when you have approximately 2 minutes left.

You are not required to examine a patient.

The encounter should be focused on the task: you will be penalised for asking irrelevant questions or providing superfluous information. You will be marked on your ability to communicate, not the speed with which you convey information. You may not have time to complete the communication.

Role: An ST4 in paediatrics.

Setting: Paediatric oncology ward.

You are talking to: Kelly Smith, a nursing student who has been working on the ward for several weeks.

Background information: One of your patients is a 12-year-old boy called Liam. He was transferred from a local district general hospital having been admitted there with a history of cough, malaise and weight loss. After further investigations, a diagnosis of leukaemia was made and he was referred to your ward for further management by the multi-disciplinary oncology team. His parents have been fully informed of the diagnosis and management, which would involve chemotherapy but carries a good prognosis, with the possibility of a cure.

Liam's parents have not told him about the diagnosis, and have asked the medical and nursing team not to tell him either, despite the fact that they have agreed to treatment. Liam was very close to his grandfather, who died of cancer last year after a prolonged period of illness, and his parents feel that it would be too upsetting for Liam to have the diagnosis discussed with him.

Kelly has looked after Liam every day since his admission. She is worried about what she should say to him, as he keeps asking about the test results and she does not want to lie to him.

She asks to speak to you about this.

Task: To discuss with Kelly her concerns about the situation and the options available to the multi-disciplinary team in dealing with it.

Points to consider:

▶ Acknowledge that this is a difficult situation, and address Kelly's concerns about telling Liam the diagnosis.

▶ Demonstrate an understanding of the role and responsibilities of a paediatrician in such a situation.

▶ Demonstrate an understanding of, and ability to discuss, the concept of Gillick competence.

▶ Demonstrate awareness that not complying with the request made by Liam's parents will risk alienating them from the multi-disciplinary team.

▶ Demonstrate awareness of possible strategies for dealing with the situation (e.g. arranging a further discussion with Liam's parents, involvement of a psychologist, etc.).

Your notes:

6: Education

(e.g. please explain the situation to the SHO so that he can deal with it)

This is a 9-minute station consisting of spoken interaction. You will have up to 2 minutes before the start of the station to read this sheet and prepare yourself. You may make notes on the paper provided.

When the bell sounds you will be invited into the examination room. Please take this instruction sheet with you. The examiner will not ask questions during the 9 minutes, but will warn you when you have approximately 2 minutes left.

You are not required to examine a patient.

The encounter should be focused on the task: you will be penalised for asking irrelevant questions or providing superfluous information. You will be marked on your ability to communicate, not the speed with which you convey information. You may not have time to complete the communication.

Role: Paediatric registrar working in a busy DGH.

Setting: Side room on the paediatric ward.

You are talking to: Francesca, an FY1 doctor who has just started on your ward this week.

Background information: You have just finished the morning ward round. You saw Henry, a 3-year-old boy who had been admitted earlier in the week with a chest infection. Henry is now well enough to be discharged home. He has DiGeorge syndrome and is well known to both this department and the tertiary paediatric hospital.

Task: Please explain the diagnosis of DiGeorge syndrome to Francesca, who has no prior knowledge of the condition.

Points to consider:

▶ DiGeorge syndrome is also known as velo-cardio-facial syndrome or Shprintzen syndrome.
▶ Briefly describe the syndrome.
  — It is rare, occurring in approximately 1 in 65 000 children.
  — It is an immunodeficiency syndrome which results from abnormal development of the third and fourth pharyngeal arches.
  — The main complications associated with the syndrome include hypocalcaemia due to hypoparathyroidism, immune defects and congenital heart defects.
▶ Genetics:
▶ 22q deletion, usually sporadic but can be autosomal dominant. Confirm using fluorescence in-situ hybridisation (FISH) studies.
▶ Clinical features (ask Francesca to describe the features observed in Henry):
  — Low-set ears.
  — Hypertelorism with downward-sloping palpebral fissures.
  — Cleft lip with or without cleft palate.
  — Micrognathia.
  — Short philtrum.
▶ Immune defects:
  — As a result of absent thymus.
  — Cell-mediated deficiency, resulting in susceptibility to fungal infections and chest infections (as seen in Henry).
▶ Management:
  — Treatment of underlying congenital heart disease.
  — Aggressive and prompt treatment of associated infections.
  — Possible bone-marrow transplants/fetal thymus implants.
▶ Confirm Francesca's understanding of a relatively complicated condition, offer sources of further information, and arrange to meet again.

Your notes:

This is a 9-minute station consisting of spoken interaction. You will have up to 2 minutes before the start of the station to read this sheet and prepare yourself. You may make notes on the paper provided.

When the bell sounds you will be invited into the examination room. Please take this instruction sheet with you. The examiner will not ask questions during the 9 minutes, but will warn you when you have approximately 2 minutes left.

You are not required to examine a patient.

The encounter should be focused on the task: you will be penalised for asking irrelevant questions or providing superfluous information. You will be marked on your ability to communicate, not the speed with which you convey information. You may not have time to complete the communication.

Role: You are a paediatric registrar on call during a night shift in a busy DGH.

Setting: Doctor's office next to the general paediatric ward.

You are talking to: Vera, the SHO on call with you that night.

Background information: Vera is an SHO with whom you have been working for the last 4 months. Earlier that evening you had been called urgently to A&E where they were treating a 4-year-old boy with presumed meningococcal septicaemia. Your consultant had been called, and the child – now stable – was transferred to the paediatric intensive-care unit. Vera had asked to speak to you. She was very upset as she had seen this child at the beginning of your shift. He had presented with coryzal symptoms, temperature and a blanching rash. Vera had thought he had a viral illness but was otherwise well, and had discharged him home.

Vera is very distressed, worried not only that she may be sued but also about her abilities as a paediatrician.

You know Vera quite well and have had no concerns about the standard of her work. You have noticed that she has seemed more quiet than usual and has phoned in sick on numerous occasions recently.

Task: Talk to Vera about the events that have taken place, and offer any guidance that you think is appropriate.

Points to consider:

- Ask Vera whether she would find it helpful to discuss what had happened that evening.
- Reassure her that she can talk to you in confidence.
- From a litigation point of view, unless you are experienced in this field, say that you feel it would be more appropriate to talk to your consultant. You can offer support by suggesting that you would talk to them for her or indeed with her.
- She can contact the MPS or the MDU for advice if she is worried.
- Confirm that you do not doubt her abilities as a paediatrician, and that neither you nor your colleagues have concerns about her. Children with meningococcal disease can deteriorate rapidly.
- Ask a general open question – is there anything else that she wishes to talk about?
- Is she finding things difficult either at home or at work?
- Would she like to meet up with you for a coffee outside work to talk things over?

Your notes:

This is a 9-minute station consisting of spoken interaction. You will have up to 2 minutes before the start of the station to read this sheet and prepare yourself. You may make notes on the paper provided.

When the bell sounds you will be invited into the examination room. Please take this instruction sheet with you. The examiner will not ask questions during the 9 minutes, but will warn you when you have approximately 2 minutes left.

You are not required to examine a patient.

The encounter should be focused on the task: you will be penalised for asking irrelevant questions or providing superfluous information. You will be marked on your ability to communicate, not the speed with which you convey information. You may not have time to complete the communication.

Role: Paediatric registrar.

Setting: Children's ward of a busy DGH.

You are talking to: Amy, a fifth-year medical student, currently attached to the paediatric department for her senior paediatric rotation.

Background information: Amy is attached to the paediatric department for 4 weeks as part of her senior rotation. She is shadowing you as you do the ward round one morning with an FY1 doctor.

You have just seen Georgia, a 3-year-old girl who has a known allergic reaction to egg. Her parents have an EpiPen for use outside hospital. Georgia was observed overnight on the children's ward after suffering from a reaction to cake she had eaten at a birthday party. EpiPen was successfully administered and her observations remained stable overnight. She is now ready for discharge home.

Amy has asked you what an EpiPen is and how you use it.

Task: Please explain to Amy what an EpiPen is and how you would explain to a parent how to administer it. (There will be a placebo pen available to aid your explanation.)

Points to consider:

▶ Make sure that you go to a room where you will not be disturbed, to ensure that the environment is conducive to learning.

▶ First check Amy's level of knowledge.

▶ An EpiPen is a pre-filled syringe containing adrenaline.

▶ We use adrenaline when a child or adult is suffering from an anaphylactic reaction.

▶ What does she understand by the term 'anaphylactic'?

▶ Anaphylaxis is an abnormal reaction to a particular substance which causes histamine to be released from the tissues, leading to either a local or widespread reaction.

▶ Anaphylactic shock is an extreme and potentially life-threatening allergic reaction. Widespread histamine release can lead to oedema, constriction of bronchioles, circulatory collapse and even death. (Go through the symptoms and signs with Amy.)

▶ Many children and adults have allergies. However, most do not require medical treatment.

▶ Explain the practicalities of administering the drug:
   — Stay calm; always shout for help, and follow BLS guidelines.
   — Remove the safety cap and place the tip on the child's thigh, holding the pen at right angles.
   — Hold the pen firmly; it automatically gives the correct dose of drug.
   — Hold for 10 seconds and remove the pen from the thigh. Massage the area for 5 seconds.
   — Note the time, and if you are outside hospital ensure that help is on the way.

▶ Always remind the parents to get a replacement EpiPen once they have used one.

▶ Confirm that Amy understands what you have told her by asking her to demonstrate the technique to you.

▶ Ask whether she has any further questions, and give her a written instruction leaflet to take away with her.

Your notes:

··

This is a 9-minute station consisting of spoken interaction. You will have up to 2 minutes before the start of the station to read this sheet and prepare yourself. You may make notes on the paper provided.

When the bell sounds you will be invited into the examination room. Please take this instruction sheet with you. The examiner will not ask questions during the 9 minutes, but will warn you when you have approximately 2 minutes left.

You are not required to examine a patient.

The encounter should be focused on the task: you will be penalised for asking irrelevant questions or providing superfluous information. You will be marked on your ability to communicate, not the speed with which you convey information. You may not have time to complete the communication.

··

Role: Paediatric registrar, working in a large DGH.

Setting: Doctor's office.

You are talking to: Eduardo Machin, a fourth-year medical student.

Background information: Eduardo has been attached to the paediatric department as part of one of his special study modules. He has come to find you because, while revising at home, he has been having some difficulty in understanding the oxygen haemoglobin curve. He has previously attended lectures covering this topic, and a basic knowledge of physiology is assumed.

> Task: Please explain the oxygen haemoglobin curve to Eduardo, and try to answer any other queries he may have.

Points to consider:
▶ Establish Eduardo's level of understanding.
▶ This is a difficult concept to understand, so start with the basics.
▶ What can you tell me about haemoglobin?
▶ Basic information: each haemoglobin molecule is made up of four subunits. Each subunit has a polypeptide chain (globin and a haem group). There are two types of polypeptide chain, alpha and beta. Adult haemoglobin, HbA, contains two alpha and two beta chains.

The haem group contains iron (Fe^{2+}), which can bind oxygen. One molecule of haemoglobin can bind four oxygen molecules, one on each subunit.

▸ Red cell physiology: each red cell is 8 μm in diameter. Red cells must maintain haemoglobin in the reduced state. The red cell must generate 2,3-diphosphoglycerate (2,3-DPG) to reversibly bind with haemoglobin.

▸ It may aid his understanding if you briefly mention the Embden-Meyerhof pathway.

▸ The oxygen-haemoglobin dissociation curve is an important tool for understanding how blood carries and releases oxygen. This curve relates the oxygen saturation and partial pressure of oxygen in the blood, and is determined by the affinity of haemoglobin for oxygen.

▸ Many different factors, such as pH, CO_2, temperature, 2,3-DPG levels and exercise, affect the saturation of haemoglobin with oxygen. The affinity of haemoglobin for oxygen is increased by decreased CO_2, decreased temperature, decreased 2,3-DPG levels and alkaline pH. This causes the curve to shift to the left.

▸ Use a diagram to show the factors which influence the affinity of haemoglobin for oxygen.

▸ Mention the Bohr effect, whereby changes in blood CO_2 levels enhance the release of oxygen from the blood to the tissues.

▸ Confirm Eduardo's understanding of what you have told him by asking him to now explain it to you.

▸ Arrange a further meeting if he is unsure of anything else, and point him in the direction of a good textbook and/or Internet resources.

Your notes:

This is a 9-minute station consisting of spoken interaction. You will have up to 2 minutes before the start of the station to read this sheet and prepare yourself. You may make notes on the paper provided.

When the bell sounds you will be invited into the examination room. Please take this instruction sheet with you. The examiner will not ask questions during the 9 minutes, but will warn you when you have approximately 2 minutes left.

You are not required to examine a patient.

The encounter should be focused on the task: you will be penalised for asking irrelevant questions or providing superfluous information. You will be marked on your ability to communicate, not the speed with which you convey information. You may not have time to complete the communication.

Role: Neonatal registrar.

Setting: Resource room attached to the neonatal unit.

You are talking to: Lucinda, a final-year medical student.

Background information: Lucinda has a keen interest in paediatrics and neonatology, and is spending part of her elective within the paediatric department. Today she joined you on your ward round. Currently on your unit are two babies. You are treating the first baby medically for necrotising enterocolitis (NEC). The second baby has returned from the tertiary surgical unit, where he has undergone surgery for the same condition. Lucinda has come to find you after the round to ask you to teach her about NEC.

> Task: Please explain to Lucinda the basics of necrotising entero-colitis and some of the associated risk factors. (You can assume that she has no previous knowledge.)

Points to consider:
- Has Lucinda ever heard of necrotising enterocolitis previously?
- Start with the basics. It is a condition which mainly affects preterm infants, although about 10% of cases are thought to occur in full-term infants. At present it is a disorder of unknown aetiology.

▶ A triad of factors are thought to be the main contributing factors:
  — hypoxic–ischaemic bowel injury
  — bacterial colonisation
  — enteral feeding.
▶ There are many other factors which are thought to lead to an increased risk:
  — umbilical vessel catheterisation (i.e. UVC, UAC)
  — early enteral feeding, in particular with hyperosmolar feeds
  — blood transfusions
  — congenital heart disease
  — very low birth weight
  — polycythaemia
  — maternal drug use.
▶ Damage occurs at a molecular level. Inflammation, necrosis of cells and haemorrhage appear to be heavily involved in the process.
▶ Nitric oxide is produced in large quantities, and it has been speculated that nitric oxide production leads to apoptosis (programmed cell death).
▶ The mainstays of treatment are stopping enteral feeds and starting IV fluids and intravenous antibiotics, and surgery if medical management fails.
▶ Possible areas for discussion are how we could prevent NEC, and future treatments.
▶ Clarify her understanding. There are vast amounts of literature on NEC, so you can guide her towards further reading if she is interested.

Your notes:

This is a 9-minute station consisting of spoken interaction. You will have up to 2 minutes before the start of the station to read this sheet and prepare yourself. You may make notes on the paper provided.

When the bell sounds you will be invited into the examination room. Please take this instruction sheet with you. The examiner will not ask questions during the 9 minutes, but will warn you when you have approximately 2 minutes left.

You are not required to examine a patient.

The encounter should be focused on the task: you will be penalised for asking irrelevant questions or providing superfluous information. You will be marked on your ability to communicate, not the speed with which you convey information. You may not have time to complete the communication.

Role: Paediatric registrar working in a busy DGH.

Setting: Small lecture theatre in the education centre attached to the hospital.

You are talking to: Lucy and Laura, both fourth-year medical students.

Background information: Lucy and Laura are currently attached to the paediatric department as part of their senior paediatric rotation. Last week one of your consultants gave a seminar to the whole group of medical students about infant feeding, primarily concentrating on breastfeeding. Lucy and Laura missed the seminar due to other commitments, and have asked you if you could spend 10 minutes going over some basic information with them. You have arranged to meet them in the education centre.

Task: Please discuss the feeding of term infants, primarily concentrating on the promoting of breastfeeding.

Points to consider:

▶ A good way to start this session would be to add some structure, and decide on the objectives. What do you hope to get out of this mini-teaching session?

- You could break it down into the advantages and disadvantages of breastfeeding. Take this a stage further and subdivide it into advantages/disadvantages for the baby and advantages/disadvantages for the mother.
- Discuss the differences between breast and formula milk.
- Use brainstorming as a method of getting the students to interact with you.
- Once you have covered the above, if you still have some time left, ask them to think of ways in which they might promote breastfeeding to new mothers.
- How could the WHO promote breastfeeding?
- Here in your local hospital, what strategies could be used to promote breastfeeding?
- Think about designing a poster to advertise and again promote breastfeeding. Discuss the previous campaign, 'Breast is best', and consider what worked. What could be improved?
- Finally, clarify the students' understanding.
- Arrange for them to meet the breastfeeding co-coordinator within the hospital if they want further information.

Your notes:

This is a 9-minute station consisting of spoken interaction. You will have up to 2 minutes before the start of the station to read this sheet and prepare yourself. You may make notes on the paper provided.

When the bell sounds you will be invited into the examination room. Please take this instruction sheet with you. The examiner will not ask questions during the 9 minutes, but will warn you when you have approximately 2 minutes left.

You are not required to examine a patient.

The encounter should be focused on the task: you will be penalised for asking irrelevant questions or providing superfluous information. You will be marked on your ability to communicate, not the speed with which you convey information. You may not have time to complete the communication.

Role: Paediatric registrar.

Setting: Doctor's office attached to the children's ward in a busy DGH.

You are talking to: Daniel, an FY1 doctor who has just started a 4-month attachment in paediatrics.

Background information: You have just finished the morning ward round with Daniel. On the ward this morning was Simon, an 11-year-old boy with Prader–Willi syndrome. He had been admitted with a viral gastroenteritis, and is now ready for discharge. At the end of the round Daniel takes you aside to say he has never heard of Prader–Willi syndrome, and would you briefly explain what it entails. You arrange to meet Daniel in the office to discuss it over coffee.

Task: Please talk to Daniel and teach him about Prader–Willi syndrome.

Points to consider:

▶ Does Daniel know anything about Prader–Willi syndrome?
▶ One possible way to structure this session would be under the following headings: genetics, clinical features, typical facies and prognosis.

- Start off with the basics, and explain the genetic abnormality. The syndrome is caused by an abnormality on the long arm of chromosome 15. The specific defect is located in bands 11–13, and therefore we express it as 15(15q11–13).
- Prader–Willi syndrome, along with another syndrome called Angelman syndrome, are two examples of an inheritance pattern known as 'imprinting.'
- In imprinting, a particular gene only expresses the copy of that gene derived from either the mother or the father.
- The active Prader–Willi gene is usually the paternal gene (i.e. that which is inherited from the father, so a deletion of the paternally derived long arm of chromosome 15 leads to Prader–Willi syndrome).
- The opposite is true for Angelman syndrome (i.e. a deletion of the maternal copy of the long arm of chromosome 15 leads to the syndrome).
- You can briefly mention *de novo* deletion and uniparental disomy.
- Next ask Daniel to describe the clinical features of Prader–Willi syndrome as seen in Simon. Write these down in the form of a table, as this makes the information easier to memorise and teach.
- Prognosis: Ask Daniel to think about the possible complications which may lead to reduced life expectancy (i.e. obesity, and cardiac and respiratory compromise).
- Confirm his understanding and arrange a further session. You could discuss Angelman syndrome next time. Ask him to do some reading at home to promote self-directed learning.

Your notes:

··

This is a 9-minute station consisting of spoken interaction. You will have up to 2 minutes before the start of the station to read this sheet and prepare yourself. You may make notes on the paper provided.

When the bell sounds you will be invited into the examination room. Please take this instruction sheet with you. The examiner will not ask questions during the 9 minutes, but will warn you when you have approximately 2 minutes left.

You are not required to examine a patient.

The encounter should be focused on the task: you will be penalised for asking irrelevant questions or providing superfluous information. You will be marked on your ability to communicate, not the speed with which you convey information. You may not have time to complete the communication.

··

Role: A paediatric specialist registrar working in a busy DGH.

Setting: Doctor's office on the paediatric ward.

You are talking to: Lucinda Jones, a third-year medical student.

Background information: Lucinda is attached to your firm. She has asked to speak to you alone as she is having difficulty understanding about screening tests. She was in an antenatal clinic last week where they were discussing '*screening for Down syndrome.*' She has asked if you would be able to go over this particular topic with her.

> Task: Please talk to Lucinda and explain the basics of screening tests and also what is involved in screening for Down syndrome.

Points to consider:

▶ What does Lucinda understand by the term 'screening'?
▶ Start with the basics, covering both primary prevention and secondary prevention.
▶ Screening tests are widely used in medicine to identify individuals who may be at high risk of suffering from the disease in question.
▶ Screening positive does not mean that you have the disease, so in the case of a woman who screens positive for Down syndrome, she

is at high risk of having a baby born with Down syndrome, but it is not 100% certain that her baby will have Down syndrome.

▶ Some of the terms that you may need to explain to Lucinda include:
— sensitivity
— specificity
— positive predictive value
— negative predictive value.

▶ Work through the following table with her:

Screening test result	Positive (i.e. affected)	Negative (i.e. unaffected)	Total
Positive	a	b	a + b
Negative	c	d	c + d
Total	a + c	b + d	a + b + c + d

▶ Specifically thinking about screening for Down syndrome, discuss the triple test, the quadruple test, nuchal translucency and the definitive test of amniocentesis.

▶ Confirm her understanding, and offer to arrange another session if she still has queries.

Your notes:

_____
_____
_____
_____
_____
_____
_____
_____
_____
_____
_____
_____
_____
_____
_____
_____
_____

This is a 9-minute station consisting of spoken interaction. You will have up to 2 minutes before the start of the station to read this sheet and prepare yourself. You may make notes on the paper provided.

When the bell sounds you will be invited into the examination room. Please take this instruction sheet with you. The examiner will not ask questions during the 9 minutes, but will warn you when you have approximately 2 minutes left.

You are not required to examine a patient.

The encounter should be focused on the task: you will be penalised for asking irrelevant questions or providing superfluous information. You will be marked on your ability to communicate, not the speed with which you convey information. You may not have time to complete the communication.

Role: A paediatric specialist registrar working in a busy DGH.

Setting: A seminar room in the academic centre.

You are talking to: A group of six stage 4 medical students.

Background information: You have been asked to lead a seminar for these six medical students on childhood obesity. Your consultant has specifically asked you to make the session as interactive as possible, and to think about ways of tackling national childhood obesity.

Task: Please outline how you will go about planning and delivering this teaching session to these six medical students. The session will last around 45 minutes in total, although this exam station lasts 9 minutes.

Points to consider:

- As with any teaching session, be well prepared.
- Think about your aims and objectives. You should at this point mention that you will link this with the medical school curriculum.
- Think about what equipment you will need, and the venue.
- It is a relatively small group, so the level of interaction should be high.
- Use brainstorming initially to get ideas among the group.

▶ Consider giving a short PowerPoint presentation on obesity to cover the 'causes of obesity.'

▶ There is no right or wrong way to answer this, but consider splitting the group into two subgroups of three students each, and giving them specific tasks to work on.

▶ Possible suggestions for small group tasks include the following:
  — Design a housing estate to help to combat childhood obesity.
  — How could a sports centre promote fitness?
  — How could supermarkets encourage healthy eating?
  — What role should schools be playing in trying to reduce the incidence of obesity?
  — What are the responsibilities of the paediatrician in tackling the increasing incidence of obesity?

▶ Give each group a specific task, asking them to brainstorm ideas and give a short presentation back to the rest of the group.

▶ Summarise and collate the feedback.

Your notes:

This is a 9-minute station consisting of spoken interaction. You will have up to 2 minutes before the start of the station to read this sheet and prepare yourself. You may make notes on the paper provided.

When the bell sounds you will be invited into the examination room. Please take this instruction sheet with you. The examiner will not ask questions during the 9 minutes, but will warn you when you have approximately 2 minutes left.

You are not required to examine a patient.

The encounter should be focused on the task: you will be penalised for asking irrelevant questions or providing superfluous information. You will be marked on your ability to communicate, not the speed with which you convey information. You may not have time to complete the communication.

Role: Paediatric registrar working in a busy DGH which has a 4-bedded intensive-care unit.

Setting: Quiet room attached to the PICU.

You are talking to: Jessica, a final-year medical student.

Background information: Jessica is attached to the intensive-care unit this week as part of her paediatric placement. On the unit is Georgina, a 2-year-old girl who has been involved in a road traffic accident. Her parents have been with her throughout her admission. Georgina has brainstem death, and this morning the decision has been made to switch off the ventilator. Georgina's parents are in agreement with the medical staff.

Jessica is upset and feels that we are 'giving up' on Georgina and not giving her a chance to recover. Your consultant has asked you to take Jessica to the quiet room to discuss this further with her.

Task: Please talk to Jessica, discuss her concerns, and explain the reasons behind switching off the ventilator.

Points to consider:

▶ Be empathic and create a supportive environment while you listen to Jessica.

▶ What does she understand about Georgina's condition?

▶ What is her understanding of *brainstem death?*

▶ Explain this to Jessica, and why it is appropriate to switch off the ventilator.

▶ It may be helpful at this stage to refer to the Royal College guidelines on withdrawing and withholding care. These are available online, and it may be something you could go over with Jessica at a later stage to further her understanding.

▶ Jessica may have very fixed ideas or beliefs. Acknowledge that there are no right and wrong feelings and that everyone will have their own opinions.

▶ In situations like this, there are very strict guidelines to adhere to, and at least two (but usually more) senior medical staff are involved in the decision making.

▶ Ensure you have answered all her underlying queries, and offer to arrange another meeting, perhaps over coffee in a less formal situation.

▶ This is a difficult situation for her to be in as a medical student, and there is support available if she feels this is necessary,

Your notes:

This is a 9-minute station consisting of spoken interaction. You will have up to 2 minutes before the start of the station to read this sheet and prepare yourself. You may make notes on the paper provided.

When the bell sounds you will be invited into the examination room. Please take this instruction sheet with you. The examiner will not ask questions during the 9 minutes, but will warn you when you have approximately 2 minutes left.

You are not required to examine a patient.

The encounter should be focused on the task: you will be penalised for asking irrelevant questions or providing superfluous information. You will be marked on your ability to communicate, not the speed with which you convey information. You may not have time to complete the communication.

Role: Paediatric registrar working in a busy DGH.

Setting: Children's outpatient department.

You are talking to: Daniel, a fourth-year medical student who is currently attached to your firm.

Background information: You have just seen John, a 12-year-old boy, along with his parents in clinic for routine follow-up. John has Wilson's disease and attends a residential school for children with specific learning needs.

Daniel is with you in clinic today and, between seeing patients, has asked you to teach him about Wilson's disease.

> Task: Please explain to Daniel about Wilson's disease, and try and answer any questions he may have.

Points to consider:

▶ Has Daniel heard of Wilson's disease and can he tell you anything about it?

▶ There is potentially quite a lot of information to convey in a short period of time. Consider the following structure:

— What is Wilson's disease?

— How is it inherited?

— What is the underlying pathology?
— How does it present?
— What are the characteristic features?
— How is the diagnosis made?
— What is the current recommended treatment?
— How is the condition managed?
— What is the course and prognosis of the disease?

▶ Ask Daniel whether he has any questions.
▶ Perhaps consider asking him to prepare a short presentation on Wilson's disease to share with the other medical students/junior doctors. This enhances self-directed learning.
▶ Refer him to the available reading material and Internet resources as appropriate.

Tip: Don't panic if you don't know the answers to all of the above sub-headings. At any point you can suggest that this is an excellent opportunity for both you and Daniel to go away and learn about the condition, each preparing a presentation to share with colleagues later that week.

Your notes:

This is a 9-minute station consisting of spoken interaction. You will have up to 2 minutes before the start of the station to read this sheet and prepare yourself. You may make notes on the paper provided.

When the bell sounds you will be invited into the examination room. Please take this instruction sheet with you. The examiner will not ask questions during the 9 minutes, but will warn you when you have approximately 2 minutes left.

You are not required to examine a patient.

The encounter should be focused on the task: you will be penalised for asking irrelevant questions or providing superfluous information. You will be marked on your ability to communicate, not the speed with which you convey information. You may not have time to complete the communication.

Role: Paediatric registrar working in a busy DGH.

Setting: Doctor's office attached to the paediatric ward.

You are talking to: Robert, a fourth-year medical student.

Background information: Robert is attached to your department for the next 6 weeks. He has asked if you would be able to spend a few minutes going over basic life support with him. They have covered this area in the third year at medical school, but he feels very unsure of the new guidelines.

Task: Please teach Robert paediatric basic life support. A mannequin has been provided with all of the necessary equipment.

Points to consider:
▶ Find out what Robert does know, and focus on the positive aspects of his knowledge.
▶ Outline the aims of today's teaching session.
▶ Focus on simplification, and highlight the fact that bystander resuscitation significantly improves outcome.
▶ From the new guidelines (which can be downloaded from www. resus.org), demonstrate the basic technique of paediatric basic life support.

- Now ask Robert to perform basic life support on the mannequin.
- Depending upon the time available and how confident he feels, it would be useful to practise a scenario with Robert.
- Summarise what you have told him and check his understanding.
- Give him the website details, or a printed copy of the new guidelines, for future reference.
- You could discuss paediatric BLS courses and APLS.

Your notes:

....

This is a 9-minute station consisting of spoken interaction. You will have up to 2 minutes before the start of the station to read this sheet and prepare yourself. You may make notes on the paper provided.

When the bell sounds you will be invited into the examination room. Please take this instruction sheet with you. The examiner will not ask questions during the 9 minutes, but will warn you when you have approximately 2 minutes left.

You are not required to examine a patient.

The encounter should be focused on the task: you will be penalised for asking irrelevant questions or providing superfluous information. You will be marked on your ability to communicate, not the speed with which you convey information. You may not have time to complete the communication.

....

Role: A paediatric specialist registrar working in a busy DGH.

Setting: The doctor's office on the children's ward.

You are talking to: Marcus and Samantha, who are two final-year medical students.

Background information: Marcus and Samantha are attached to your firm for the next 6 weeks. They have completed their attachment in paediatrics and have chosen to do a 'special study module' in paediatrics, as they are both interested in pursuing a career in paediatrics once they are qualified.

> Task: Please talk to Marcus and Samantha about audit. Your consultant has asked you to talk to them and agree an audit they could perform over the next 6 weeks. You can assume neither of them has any prior experience of audit.

Points to consider:

▶ What is audit?
▶ Use brainstorming as a method to both break the ice and generate ideas.
▶ There are many different definitions of audit. Make sure that you understand the difference between audit and research and are able to explain this.

▶ 'Audit is an examination or review that establishes the extent to which a condition, process or performance conforms to predetermined standards or criteria.'

▶ We need to ask ourselves the following questions. Have we any agreed aims in medical practice? If so, are we falling short of these aims?

▶ Get them to think together of some possible audit topics.

▶ There are six main stages involved in any audit:
  1. Aim (i.e. choice of topic).
  2. Setting/defining your standards.
  3. Observing current practice.
  4. Comparing performance with targets.
  5. Implementing changes.
  6. Evaluation and re-audit to complete the cycle.

▶ Possible audit topics could include meningitis guidelines, NICE guidelines for the management of the fitting child, NICE guidelines for the management of the feverish child, etc.

▶ Set a realistic timescale with them, getting them to take the lead and responsibility, as this will be good practice for the future. However, you can assist them.

▶ Closing the meeting: ensure that they have a clear understanding and that each of them understands the tasks allocated to them.

Your notes:

....

This is a 9-minute station consisting of spoken interaction. You will have up to 2 minutes before the start of the station to read this sheet and prepare yourself. You may make notes on the paper provided.

When the bell sounds you will be invited into the examination room. Please take this instruction sheet with you. The examiner will not ask questions during the 9 minutes, but will warn you when you have approximately 2 minutes left.

You are not required to examine a patient.

The encounter should be focused on the task: you will be penalised for asking irrelevant questions or providing superfluous information. You will be marked on your ability to communicate, not the speed with which you convey information. You may not have time to complete the communication.

....

Role: A paediatric specialist registrar working in a busy DGH.

Setting: Seminar room in the education centre.

You are talking to: A group of 8 final-year medical students.

Background information: These 8 medical students are attached to your paediatric department for a month as part of their final-year senior rotations. They have asked you if you would be able to go over some specific topics with them, which they are all having trouble understanding. The topic you have chosen today is *evidence-based medicine (EBM)*.

Task: Please explain to these students what EBM is and its relevance to clinical medicine.

Points to consider:

▶ Think of your setting. You have a relatively small group of 8 students here, so possible teaching methods would include 'round robin', brainstorming as a group using a flip chart, working initially in pairs and then each pair feeding back to the group.
▶ What is evidence-based medicine?
▶ Get the students to come up with their own ideas, and make the session as interactive as possible.

▶ There are many definitions, the most commonly known being that taken from David Sackett: 'the conscientious, explicit and judicious use of current best evidence in making decisions about the care of the individual patient.'
▶ Pose questions to the students – for example, do we all as clinicians have a responsibility to take part in EBM?
▶ There are six main stages involved:
  — You are faced with a clinical problem from the care of an individual patient.
  — From this you are able to define a question.
  — Search for the latest evidence.
  — Is this evidence applicable to your patient?
  — Consider the evidence, your clinical expertise and patient preferences.
  — Evaluate all the above knowledge and formulate an individual care plan for your patient.
▶ Finally, work through some 'real' clinical examples – for example, 'Should steroids be used in the treatment of viral induced wheeze in children?'
▶ Mention the Cochrane database, NICE and CHI.

Your notes:

This is a 9-minute station consisting of spoken interaction. You will have up to 2 minutes before the start of the station to read this sheet and prepare yourself. You may make notes on the paper provided.

When the bell sounds you will be invited into the examination room. Please take this instruction sheet with you. The examiner will not ask questions during the 9 minutes, but will warn you when you have approximately 2 minutes left.

You are not required to examine a patient.

The encounter should be focused on the task: you will be penalised for asking irrelevant questions or providing superfluous information. You will be marked on your ability to communicate, not the speed with which you convey information. You may not have time to complete the communication.

Role: Paediatric registrar working in a busy DGH.

Setting: Side room on the paediatric ward.

You are talking to: Jacob, one of a group of fourth-year medical students.

Background information: Jacob is one of six medical students currently attached to your ward as part of their paediatric rotation. On the ward round you have just seen a 4-year-old girl with an exacerbation of asthma. Jacob asks to talk to you after the round. He had heard that the incidence of asthma was increasing and that this was thought to be due to excessive cleanliness. He had not understood what was meant by this statement.

Task: Please talk to Jacob about the 'hygiene hypothesis' and how this is related to asthma.

Points to consider:

 Brainstorm the idea that Jacob has raised with him. Get him to think about what it may be implying and the consequences that this would have if true.

 The hypothesis he is referring to, known as the 'hygiene hypothesis', is a fairly new school of thought which argues that the rising incidence of not only asthma but also other conditions such as inflammatory bowel disease and multiple sclerosis may at least in part be the result of changes in our immune system.

▶ One proposed theory for these immune system changes is the result of lifestyle and environmental changes that have made us 'too clean.'

▶ What lifestyle and environmental changes can Jacob think of which may have led to this situation?

▶ It has been suggested that improved hygiene and a lack of exposure to micro-organisms may be affecting the immune system, particularly in individuals who live in developed countries.

▶ This is making individuals more susceptible to certain diseases, including autoimmune disease.

▶ A paper was published in January 2005 which stated that these were inconsistent findings and were unlikely to be the sole explanation for the ongoing asthma epidemic.

▶ This hygiene hypothesis is mentioned in the British Asthma Guidelines.

▶ As a way of promoting self-directed learning, suggest that Jacob does an Internet search for any literature, and then shares his findings with you and the rest of the group.

Your notes:

....

This is a 6-minute station. You will have 3 minutes beforehand to read this sheet and prepare yourself. You may take the sheet with you into the station, but you must return it at the end.

....

Role: A GP.

Setting: Your surgery.

You are talking to: A final-year medical student.

Background information: You have just seen an 8-month-old baby with bronchiolitis. The medical student was present during the consultation. You have given advice to the baby's mother and her partner about the condition and arranged a review as appropriate.

Task: To teach the medical student about bronchiolitis, emphasising the indications for hospital referral.

YOU ARE NOT EXPECTED TO GATHER THE REST OF THE MEDICAL HISTORY DURING THIS CONSULTATION.

Points to consider:

▶ Enquire about the medical student's main concerns regarding this case. He appears keen to learn. Acknowledge this. He may be worried that the infant needs to be admitted to hospital.
▶ Ascertain the student's knowledge base about bronchiolitis.
▶ Give a simple explanation of the features of bronchiolitis and the indications for referral, such as poor feeding, cyanosis, marked tachypnoea, apnoea, high temperature, significant breathing difficulties, and parents' inability to cope or the presence of other social issues.
▶ Confirm that there is no role for antibiotics/bronchodilators or steroids in bronchiolitis.
▶ Summarise what you have told the student.
▶ Check his understanding as you give him the information, and afterwards.
▶ Offer him a useful resource, such as reading material, and website or hospital/local guidelines.

Your notes:

7: Difficult conversations/ other

Role: Paediatric specialist registrar working in a DGH.

Setting: Clinic room of a general paediatric outpatient department.

You are talking to: Mrs Maddison, mother of 15-month-old Lewis.

Background information: Lewis has attended his GP surgery with an ear infection in the past 12 months, but has no other medical problems. He was due to have his MMR vaccination, but his mother did not attend. She has since seen her GP and asked for a referral to outpatients so that she can discuss MMR vaccines in further detail.

Task: Discuss with Mrs Maddison her concerns regarding the MMR vaccine.

Points to consider:

▶ Thank Mrs Maddison for coming to see you today, say that you understand she has some concerns about the MMR vaccine, and invite her to discuss them.

▶ You may need to structure the conversation. One possible structure to think about would be to first talk a bit about the actual vaccine itself. Live attenuated vaccine contains weakened versions of live measles, mumps and rubella viruses. Because the viruses are weakened, people who have recently had the vaccine cannot infect other people.

▶ Next discuss its effectiveness. It is highly effective, and has almost wiped out the three diseases since it was introduced in the UK in 1988.

▶ Side-effects: mention local, minor effects of fever, redness, rash and swollen glands.

▶ Others side-effects which parents may mention include 'fever fits' and sub-acute sclerosing pan-encephalitis (SSPE).

▶ The issues that cause greatest concern are the links between MMR and autism and between MMR and bowel problems.

▶ Acknowledge Mrs Maddison's concerns. There have been many stories in the media linking MMR with these conditions, and you can understand why she is confused.

▶ You accept that this is her decision whether to vaccinate her child. You are not there to make the decision for her, but simply to provide her with the information that will enable her to make an informed choice.

▶ You would recommend that all children (unless there are genuine medical contraindications) should receive the MMR vaccine.

▶ Independent medical experts from around the world have found no link between MMR and autism and bowel problems.

▶ The Medical Research Council and the Committee on Safety of Medicines state that the use of separate vaccines may be harmful.

▶ Finally summarise what you have told her, check her understanding and offer written information, or refer her to the Department of Health website.

Your notes:

This is a 9-minute station consisting of spoken interaction. You will have up to 2 minutes before the start of the station to read this sheet and prepare yourself. You may make notes on the paper provided.

When the bell sounds you will be invited into the examination room. Please take this instruction sheet with you. The examiner will not ask questions during the 9 minutes, but will warn you when you have approximately 2 minutes left.

You are not required to examine a patient.

The encounter should be focused on the task: you will be penalised for asking irrelevant questions or providing superfluous information. You will be marked on your ability to communicate, not the speed with which you convey information. You may not have time to complete the communication.

Role: Paediatric registrar working in a busy DGH.

Setting: Side room on the children's ward.

You are talking to: Miss Waters, 19-year-old mother of Corey, who is 5 weeks old.

Background information: Corey was born at 34 weeks' gestation via normal delivery after spontaneous preterm labour. He was well at birth and did not require any resuscitation. He spent 3 weeks on the neonatal unit. Nursing staff on the unit had some concerns about Miss Waters; she would visit at erratic times and comment that she could not bond with Corey. Social services were involved and Corey was discharged home with follow-up arranged. During a routine visit by his health visitor she was concerned that Corey had some bruising around his mouth, and had arranged for him to be brought to A&E.

The A&E registrar has seen Corey and is worried about non-accidental injury. He has asked you to take over Corey's care.

Task: Please discuss these issues with Miss Waters, and outline your immediate management plan.

Points to consider:

▶ When dealing with cases of non-accidental injury, be honest and open with the parents/carers.

▶ Do not pass judgment or blame the parents/carers, as this is not your responsibility. Always involve senior colleagues if you have little experience.

▶ Ask Miss Waters if she knows why the A&E staff have asked you to review Corey.

▶ Does she have any idea how he got the bruises?

▶ Concentrate on the immediate management of Corey.

▶ Highlight the need to keep Corey safe, and follow the hospital protocol with regard to necessary investigations.

▶ Explain the relevant investigations to exclude medical conditions which may have led to the bruising.

▶ Social services will need to be informed. Again emphasise that this is to make sure the home environment is safe for Cory.

▶ The conversation may be difficult if Miss Waters becomes angry or upset. Remain calm, ask for help when necessary, and again highlight the fact that Corey's health is your priority.

▶ Summarise, and allow ample time for questions.

Your notes:

This is a 9-minute station consisting of spoken interaction. You will have up to 2 minutes before the start of the station to read this sheet and prepare yourself. You may make notes on the paper provided.

When the bell sounds you will be invited into the examination room. Please take this instruction sheet with you. The examiner will not ask questions during the 9 minutes, but will warn you when you have approximately 2 minutes left.

You are not required to examine a patient.

The encounter should be focused on the task: you will be penalised for asking irrelevant questions or providing superfluous information. You will be marked on your ability to communicate, not the speed with which you convey information. You may not have time to complete the communication.

Role: Neonatal registrar working in a busy district general hospital.

Setting: Side room on the central delivery suite.

You are talking to: Lisa Teller, a first-year midwifery student.

Background information: You have just attended a delivery at which Lisa was present. Baby Joseph Moss was born by normal vaginal delivery at 38 weeks' gestation. Antenatally, a diagnosis of hypoplastic left heart was made. His parents were counselled and the treatment options were outlined. They visited the tertiary cardiac centre and spoke to the cardiac team who would be involved in caring for Joseph. Throughout the pregnancy the parents were in regular contact with the cardiac liaison sister and the obstetric team. His parents made the decision not to pursue any treatment once Joseph was born. They fully understood the decision they had made and asked that Joseph be kept comfortable after birth. They requested that they as a family could spend whatever time they had with Joseph.

Lisa is very distressed and has asked to talk to you. She feels that we are letting Joseph die, and that perhaps his parents do not realise he could have surgery to save his life.

Task: Please talk to Lisa about her concerns and give her some further information about hypoplastic left heart syndrome.

Points to consider:

- Meet with Lisa in private, somewhere where you will not be interrupted.
- You need to acknowledge this is obviously a distressing issue for her to talk about.
- Start by exploring exactly what knowledge she has about congenital heart disease, in particular hypoplastic left heart syndrome.
- Go back to basics, assuming no prior knowledge.
- It is often a good idea to draw a very basic diagram of the heart at this stage, as it makes explaining the diagnosis much easier when you can visualise it.
- It is a spectrum of disorders where the aortic and mitral valve and the left ventricle are too small and under-developed to maintain a systemic output. Use your diagram to help to explain each of these in turn.
- Around 200–400 babies are born with this condition each year in the UK.
- There are two main surgical options: Norwood two-stage procedure or heart transplantation.
- Explain that both of the surgical options are major operations and carry significant risks of morbidity and mortality. You do not need to go into great detail about the procedures themselves.
- Even if Joseph had surgical correction, he would not have a 'normal heart', and he would have many years of both surgical and medical intervention ahead of him.
- Joseph's parents have had the full support of the tertiary cardiac unit in making their decision, and we must now respect that decision even if we do not agree with it.
- Admire the fact that she is thinking of these issues, and emphasise how important it is to be the child's advocate and to ensure that the families of these children have had every opportunity to make fully informed decisions.
- Ensure that you have covered all of the issues she wants to raise, offer to meet again if she has further questions, and also offer her further information (e.g. from Internet resources) about these heart conditions and the various options and support available.

Your notes:

This is a 9-minute station consisting of spoken interaction. You will have up to 2 minutes before the start of the station to read this sheet and prepare yourself. You may make notes on the paper provided.

When the bell sounds you will be invited into the examination room. Please take this instruction sheet with you. The examiner will not ask questions during the 9 minutes, but will warn you when you have approximately 2 minutes left.

You are not required to examine a patient.

The encounter should be focused on the task: you will be penalised for asking irrelevant questions or providing superfluous information. You will be marked on your ability to communicate, not the speed with which you convey information. You may not have time to complete the communication.

Role: Neonatal registrar.

Setting: Side room on the neonatal unit.

You are talking to: Mrs Banks, mother of 48-hour-old Josie.

Background information: Josie was born at term via a forceps delivery after an uneventful pregnancy. She had been well until about 12 hours of age, when she became lethargic, pyrexial and could not tolerate feeds. She was transferred from the postnatal ward to the neonatal intensive-care unit. Blood cultures taken at the time of admission to the unit have grown group B streptococcus. Josie is intubated and ventilated and requiring inotropic support. Her parents have been kept fully updated about her condition.

Mrs Banks has come round to the unit demanding to speak to a doctor. She is angry and upset because someone has told her that she should have been tested while she was pregnant for the bug that has made Josie unwell.

Task: Please take Mrs Banks into the relative's room and talk to her about her concerns.

Points to consider:
▶ Try to take control of the situation by calming Mrs Banks down,

acknowledging that she is obviously upset, and reassuring her that you can take time to discuss her concerns.

▶ What does she understand by 'Group B streptococcus infection'?

▶ Give some brief basic information. Group B streptococcus is a bug, or micro-organism, which can cause serious infection in a newborn baby. There are two usual patterns – that of early onset (presenting in the first week, mostly within 3 days after birth), which is seen in about 80% of babies, and that of late onset (after about 7 days of age), which is seen in the remaining 20% of babies.

▶ In about 1 in 4–5 healthy pregnant women the GBS organism is present in the vagina or rectal region at term. This does not cause any problems to pregnant mothers, but a small number (less than 1%) of babies can develop early-onset disease.

▶ As far as you understand it is not our practice to perform routine screening for GBS on all pregnant mothers. However, this is an obstetric issue and therefore you do not feel that you are the best person to deal with this concern.

▶ Concentrate on Josie. At present you are treating her with antibiotics and supporting her heart and breathing.

▶ This is a very difficult time for Mrs Banks. Josie is seriously unwell, but everything possible is being done for her at the present time.

▶ Offer to arrange a joint meeting between yourselves and the obstetric team, as they may be able to address her needs more appropriately.

▶ Encourage her to come to the unit to see Josie, and offer your full support.

▶ Arrange a further meeting to keep her updated on Josie's progress, and tell her that you will inform your consultant and the obstetric team about her concerns.

Your notes:

This is a 9-minute station consisting of spoken interaction. You will have up to 2 minutes before the start of the station to read this sheet and prepare yourself. You may make notes on the paper provided.

When the bell sounds you will be invited into the examination room. Please take this instruction sheet with you. The examiner will not ask questions during the 9 minutes, but will warn you when you have approximately 2 minutes left.

You are not required to examine a patient.

The encounter should be focused on the task: you will be penalised for asking irrelevant questions or providing superfluous information. You will be marked on your ability to communicate, not the speed with which you convey information. You may not have time to complete the communication.

Role: Paediatric registrar.

Setting: Outpatient clinic in a busy DGH.

You are talking to: Mrs Rahman, mother of 8-week-old Ranjeet.

Background information: Ranjeet was born at 37 weeks' gestation via normal delivery after an uneventful pregnancy. He has been referred to you by his GP with concerns regarding excessive crying. On examination the GP found Ranjeet to be a healthy baby who is gaining weight and is developmentally age appropriate. His main concern is that Mrs Rahman is feeding Ranjeet on goat's milk and is considering starting him on solids. Mrs Rahman has three other children, all healthy, aged 2, 4 and 5 years. Mr Rahman no longer lives with the family.

Task: Please discuss Mrs Rahman's concerns about Ranjeet's excessive crying, and advise her against both using goat's milk and starting him on solids.

Points to consider:

▶ Briefly go over the pregnancy. Was it planned? Were the scans normal? Was Mrs Rahman well during pregnancy?
▶ Now go over the delivery. What was the mode of delivery? Did she receive support during delivery and immediately afterwards?

▶ Enquire about the excessive crying.

▶ What are her main concerns and worries?

▶ Reassure her that the GP has examined Ranjeet and thinks he is doing very well – offer praise here. You do not think there is a physical reason for his excessive crying.

▶ Take a detailed feeding history. What was the reason for changing to goat's milk?

▶ *Do not blame or accuse her*, but explain that goat's milk and cow's milk are not suitable for babies until 12 months of age. This is because they have insufficient amounts of vitamins and iron and contain too much protein and salt.

▶ Be empathic – it must be very difficult and exhausting for her with four small children at home.

▶ Is there anyone at home who supports her? Any friends or relatives?

▶ Again explain that the WHO advises against feeding solids until 6 months of age. Give the reasons for this.

▶ Try to reach a compromise, formulate a management plan, agree on a suitable formula milk, and plan a routine for Ranjeet. Put Mrs Rahman in touch with local services that offer further support (e.g. health visitor, sure start, local mother and toddler groups).

▶ Arrange follow-up to see how things are progressing.

▶ Confirm her understanding and ask whether she has any other issues that you may be able to help her with.

Your notes:

This is a 9-minute station consisting of spoken interaction. You will have up to 2 minutes before the start of the station to read this sheet and prepare yourself. You may make notes on the paper provided.

When the bell sounds you will be invited into the examination room. Please take this instruction sheet with you. The examiner will not ask questions during the 9 minutes, but will warn you when you have approximately 2 minutes left.

You are not required to examine a patient.

The encounter should be focused on the task: you will be penalised for asking irrelevant questions or providing superfluous information. You will be marked on your ability to communicate, not the speed with which you convey information. You may not have time to complete the communication.

Role: Neonatal registrar.

Setting: Side room on the neonatal intensive-care unit.

You are talking to: Gill Firth, senior midwife and breastfeeding liaison sister.

Background information: Gill has come round to the neonatal unit from the postnatal ward to speak to you about Molly Sanders, a 5-day-old baby girl who is currently on the ward with her mother. Molly is jaundiced and not breastfeeding very well. Your SHO has been to review Molly this morning and arranged to do a blood test. He had told the mother that Molly will need to be cared for on the neonatal unit and will most probably need formula feeds. Gill is upset about this, as she feels that we do not give these babies a chance to establish breast-feeding, and taking them to the NICU disrupts the mother–baby bond. Apart from the jaundice, Molly is otherwise healthy.

Task: Please discuss with Gill what her concerns are, and how they can best be resolved.

Points to consider:

▶ First gather some more information. You need to know about Molly's history and the exchange of information that occurred that morning.

▶ Listen to Gill and explore the issues that have upset her.

▶ You should promote breastfeeding, but at the same time you must ensure the health of the child.

▶ The only way for you to accurately assess whether Molly needs to be cared for on the neonatal unit is to examine Molly yourself, so offer to do this.

▶ Communication with the mother is also vital.

▶ Explore the possible reasons for poor feeding. Is there an underlying medical condition which has been overlooked?

▶ What are the mother's feelings about feeding?

▶ What has been tried so far to promote feeding?

▶ If supplemental feeding is considered to be necessary, what are the options? Consider nasogastric feeds, syringe feeds and cup feeds.

▶ Consider expressed breast milk as opposed to formula feeds.

▶ Make sure that you have agreed a way forward with Gill and Molly's mother before you leave. It may be that a further team meeting between neonatal staff and midwifery staff needs to be arranged to aid communication and team building in future.

▶ Ensure that you have covered all of the issues which Gill feels are important, and thank her for raising them with you.

Your notes:

This is a 9-minute station consisting of spoken interaction. You will have up to 2 minutes before the start of the station to read this sheet and prepare yourself. You may make notes on the paper provided.

When the bell sounds you will be invited into the examination room. Please take this instruction sheet with you. The examiner will not ask questions during the 9 minutes, but will warn you when you have approximately 2 minutes left.

You are not required to examine a patient.

The encounter should be focused on the task: you will be penalised for asking irrelevant questions or providing superfluous information. You will be marked on your ability to communicate, not the speed with which you convey information. You may not have time to complete the communication.

Role: Paediatric registrar working in a busy DGH.

Setting: Children's outpatient clinic.

You are talking to: Mr David Bennett, a school nurse.

Background information: Mr Bennett is a school nurse from the local secondary school, where Matthew, one of your patients, attends. Matthew is a 15-year-old boy who has cystic fibrosis. Mr Bennett contacted your consultant to ask for an appointment to see him to discuss Matthew, as he is concerned about both his attendance and his behaviour at school.

Matthew's parents are aware of the appointment and are grateful for the support they receive from Mr Bennett.

Task: Please meet Mr Bennett and address his concerns about Matthew.

Points to consider:

▶ Thank Mr Bennett for coming to meet with you today.
▶ You understand that he has some concerns about Matthew. Would he like to discuss these concerns?
▶ It may be that you need to lead the conversation. Perhaps consider structuring it under the following headings:

- — What is Mr Bennett's understanding of cystic fibrosis?
- — Explain the basics of cystic fibrosis, highlighting the fact that it is a genetic, incurable condition.
- — Management: pharmacological and physiotherapy.
- — Course and prognosis – life expectancy.
- — Significant psychological impact on both the child and their family.
- — The need for repeated hospital visits, both as an inpatient and for clinic appointments.
- — School: attendance, academic progress, friendships, possible difficulties with PE or travel to school, being different from his peer group.

▶ Suggest that it may be helpful to arrange a multi-disciplinary meeting involving the school, Matthew, his parents and health professionals in order to provide Matthew and his parents with a greater level of support.

▶ Arrange to discuss this with Matthew's consultant, and offer to contact his parents.

▶ Give Mr Bennett an opportunity to ask questions.

▶ Make suitable arrangements for contacting Mr Bennett in the near future.

Your notes:

This is a 9-minute station consisting of spoken interaction. You will have up to 2 minutes before the start of the station to read this sheet and prepare yourself. You may make notes on the paper provided.

When the bell sounds you will be invited into the examination room. Please take this instruction sheet with you. The examiner will not ask questions during the 9 minutes, but will warn you when you have approximately 2 minutes left.

You are not required to examine a patient.

The encounter should be focused on the task: you will be penalised for asking irrelevant questions or providing superfluous information. You will be marked on your ability to communicate, not the speed with which you convey information. You may not have time to complete the communication.

Role: Paediatric registrar working in a busy DGH.

Setting: Children's outpatient clinic.

You are talking to: Hayley Young, a 15-year-old girl with cystic fibrosis.

Background information: Hayley is well known to your department, and she has attended with her mother this morning. There has been a sudden deterioration in her lung function. Previously Hayley has always been compliant with both medication and hospital visits.

She has asked to speak to you alone.

Task: Please see Hayley and explore any concerns that she has, trying to find an explanation for her recent deterioration in lung function.

Points to consider:

▶ The most important factor in this station will be building a rapport with Hayley.

▶ As this is the first time you have met her, ask her whether it would be all right to briefly ask her some questions in order to get to know her a bit better. This gives her the opportunity to relax and gain trust in you.

▶ A suggested structure for your conversation might be as follows:
— Recap briefly on her history: age at diagnosis, hospital admissions.
— Take a current history, including symptoms in the last few weeks or months. Has she been well/unwell?
— Explore her usual medication and physiotherapy regime (compliance).
— School situation: academic progress, friends, peer group, boyfriends/relationships, bullying.
— Social factors: smoking, alcohol, recreational drug use, sexual relationships.
— Home situation: relationship with parents/siblings, support.
— Are there any particular issues which Hayley is finding hard to deal with or would like to talk about?

▶ This may be a problem of compliance. However, there could equally well be a genuine medical reason for her decline in lung function, so avoid being judgmental. This will help to build rapport.

▶ Thank Hayley for being honest with you, and acknowledge that it must have been difficult for her to talk to you today.

▶ Close by agreeing a way forward with her, which may involve an increased level of support, involving specialist CF nurses or the school nurse, or arranging to see her again in clinic.

Your notes:

This is a 9-minute station consisting of spoken interaction. You will have up to 2 minutes before the start of the station to read this sheet and prepare yourself. You may make notes on the paper provided.

When the bell sounds you will be invited into the examination room. Please take this instruction sheet with you. The examiner will not ask questions during the 9 minutes, but will warn you when you have approximately 2 minutes left.

You are not required to examine a patient.

The encounter should be focused on the task: you will be penalised for asking irrelevant questions or providing superfluous information. You will be marked on your ability to communicate, not the speed with which you convey information. You may not have time to complete the communication.

Role: Paediatric registrar working in a busy DGH.

Setting: Children's outpatient clinic.

You are talking to: Mark, a 15-year-old boy with type 1 diabetes.

Background information: Mark has had diabetes for the last 4 years, and has previously been well controlled and compliant with medication and hospital attendances. His GP has requested an early review in clinic because he is concerned about the recent deterioration in Mark's blood sugar control. He has also had a recent admission with diabetic ketoacidosis. His mother is worried that he has recently become quiet and withdrawn, spending long periods of time alone in his bedroom.

Mark has asked to speak to you alone.

Task: Please speak to Mark, and explore the possible reasons for his recent deterioration in blood sugar control.

Points to consider:

▶ Start by asking Mark if he knows why his GP has asked for him to be seen today.
▶ Consider the following structure as a way of gaining his trust and building rapport so that he feels able to confide in you:

- — Do you remember when you were first diagnosed? Can you tell me a little bit about that time?
- — What was your initial reaction? How did you cope with the diagnosis, injections, glucose monitoring and diet?
- — How did your family/friends respond (education package)?
- — Current treatment regime.
- — Monitoring and control of blood sugar.
- — School: academic progress, friends, bullying, support, attendance.
- — Social: smoking, alcohol, recreational drug use, independence.
▶ Introduce the reason why he is here. Your GP is concerned that your control is perhaps not as good as it used to be. Also mention the recent admission for DKA.
▶ Can he think of any triggers which might be responsible?
- — Insulin compliance.
- — Appetite, general health, weight loss/gain.
- — Sleep pattern, exercise.
▶ Acknowledge that diabetes is a difficult condition to live with, especially when you are a teenager. Address the psychological component.
▶ Reiterate why tight control of his blood sugar level is so important.
▶ Does he have any particular underlying worries?
▶ Would he benefit from some extra support (e.g. input at school, meeting other young people with diabetes, education session, camps, and activity days)?
▶ Arrange a review appointment and provide contact telephone numbers for support.

Your notes:

This is a 9-minute station consisting of spoken interaction. You will have up to 2 minutes before the start of the station to read this sheet and prepare yourself. You may make notes on the paper provided.

When the bell sounds you will be invited into the examination room. Please take this instruction sheet with you. The examiner will not ask questions during the 9 minutes, but will warn you when you have approximately 2 minutes left.

You are not required to examine a patient.

The encounter should be focused on the task: you will be penalised for asking irrelevant questions or providing superfluous information. You will be marked on your ability to communicate, not the speed with which you convey information. You may not have time to complete the communication.

Role: Paediatric registrar working in a busy DGH.

Setting: Side room of the adolescent bay, attached to the children's ward.

You are talking to: Lucas, a 15-year-old boy.

Background information: Lucas was admitted to the ward via A&E in the early hours of this morning. He had been found drunk in a park, after his friends had called the police. There were no other injuries. Lucas was admitted to the ward and received IV fluids overnight. Apart from a headache he is well this morning and ready for discharge home. His parents have been contacted and his father will be collecting him shortly.

Task: Please discuss the admission with Lucas, in particular highlighting the dangers of drug and alcohol ingestion in young people.

Points to consider:

▶ One of the most important factors here is to establish rapport with Lucas.
▶ Although his behaviour was inappropriate and immature, you need to treat him with respect and discuss the important issues.

▶ Start off with open questions. How does he feel this morning about the incident last night?

▶ Try to engage him, and highlight the potential dangers of excess alcohol.

▶ You may also wish to mention recreational drug use, smoking and risky behaviour.

▶ How does he think his parents will react?

▶ Does he drink on a regular basis? If he does, it may be appropriate to suggest a referral to the drugs and alcohol service for young people.

▶ You need to ascertain whether this was a 'one-off' incident or a regular pattern of behaviour, perhaps due to peer pressure.

▶ Offer support, while at the same time being clear and firm about just how serious and dangerous this incident could have been.

▶ Finally, ask whether there are any underlying issues that he wishes to discuss with you. You may want to enquire about his home circumstances, friends and school.

▶ Arrange follow-up or offer to speak to his parents if appropriate.

▶ Offer him the contact telephone numbers of support groups if appropriate.

Your notes:

This is a 9-minute station consisting of spoken interaction. You will have up to 2 minutes before the start of the station to read this sheet and prepare yourself. You may make notes on the paper provided.

When the bell sounds you will be invited into the examination room. Please take this instruction sheet with you. The examiner will not ask questions during the 9 minutes, but will warn you when you have approximately 2 minutes left.

You are not required to examine a patient.

The encounter should be focused on the task: you will be penalised for asking irrelevant questions or providing superfluous information. You will be marked on your ability to communicate, not the speed with which you convey information. You may not have time to complete the communication.

Role: Paediatric registrar working in a DGH.

Setting: Cubicle on the neonatal unit.

You are talking to: Mrs Gilmore, mother of 3-week-old Robbie.

Background information: Robbie was born at 35 weeks' gestation after a difficult pregnancy. He had an antenatal diagnosis of gastroschisis, and was transferred to the regional paediatric surgical centre. He underwent repair and has made good progress. He has been transferred back to his local hospital for continuing care.

Routine admission swabs have isolated MRSA. This has been discussed with the microbiologist and your consultant, and although Robbie is well, the decision has been made to commence eradication treatment.

Task: Please inform Mrs Gilmore of the diagnosis and expected management plan.

Points to consider:

▶ This could potentially be a very difficult conversation with an angry and/or upset mother.
▶ You need to remain calm and in control of the situation, and reassure Mrs Gilmore that you appreciate this is a very difficult time for her.

- Set the scene for her by explaining why you have been asked to come and talk to her.
- Routine swabs are always taken on any baby who is transferred to your unit from another hospital. This is to try to prevent the spread of infection.
- Robbie is very well in himself. However, the skin swabs have grown a bug called MRSA.
- Mrs Gilmore will probably be alarmed at the mention of MRSA, as most parents interpret this as the 'superbug', and she is likely to be visibly upset and angry.
- Allow her time to express her emotions. Remain very calm and explain that you are going to go through what this means for Robbie and the management plan.
- She may ask 'Is he going to die?'. This is a difficult question to answer, but you must be honest. It is unlikely, as Robbie is very well, he will be closely monitored, and some treatment will be started to try to eradicate the bug. However, there is a risk associated with every infection that a baby may become more unwell.
- Explain how important *handwashing* is, and the reasons for this.
- If you are able to contain the situation, clarify her understanding and ask whether she has any further questions.
- It may be that you need to arrange for her to meet with Robbie's consultant to discuss this further.

Your notes:

Role: A GP registrar.

Setting: GP surgery.

You are talking to: Hannah, the mother of 13-week-old infant, Rain.

Background information: Rain was born at term gestation by a normal vaginal delivery. She has never settled. She cries all the time, both day and night. She does not settle with feeds, and is occasionally sick after feeds. The health visitor changed her milk formula 5 weeks ago, but without any improvement. She continues to grow along the 75th centile for weight. She has had a number of visits so far to her GP and the A&E department. She has been treated for gastro-oesophageal reflux and constipation for 2 weeks without any response.

Examination is essentially normal. Both parents are exhausted due to constant sleepless nights with Rain.

Other information: The mother and father are 17 and 19 years old, respectively, and are not receiving any help from extended family. Both are unemployed and on income support. They are angry and upset about having to visit the hospital/GP surgery so often, all to no avail.

Task: To explain to the mother your suspicion of cow's milk protein intolerance, and the need to stop all medications and the trial of special formula milk.

YOU ARE NOT EXPECTED TO GATHER THE REST OF THE MEDICAL HISTORY DURING THIS CONSULTATION.

Points to consider:

▶ Explore the mother's specific concerns about Rain's condition. She may be anxious about Rain having a serious problem with her tummy, or unhappy that the medications are not working and no tests have been carried out so far to confirm a diagnosis. She may be very tired due to not having had any sleep for several nights. She may want Rain to be admitted to hospital for proper care. Gaining a better insight into the mother's concerns will help you to offer specific advice and win her confidence.

▶ Explain the diagnosis of cow's milk protein intolerance.

▶ Reassure the mother that there is no evidence to suggest that there are any serious abnormalities of the gut.

▶ Acknowledge the parent's worries, but reassure her using the growth parameters.

▶ Explain that this is a trial to determine what the effects of the special formula are, and whether it would be better for Rain to avoid cow's milk.

▶ Arrange for regular reviews to monitor Rain's progress.

▶ Offer support from a health visitor and social services as necessary.

Your notes:

This is a 6-minute station. You will have 3 minutes beforehand to read this sheet and prepare yourself. You may take the sheet with you into the station, but you must return it at the end.

Role: A GP registrar.

Setting: GP surgery.

You are talking to: Your GP colleague (male or female).

Background information: You have just seen Vicky, a single mother with two young children, Dixie, aged 2 years, and Angela, aged 10 months. Vicky came to see you with a non-specific rash. She brought both children with her.

The children were unwashed, filthy and wearing dirty clothes. They were very clingy, but were happy to play in the waiting room. Vicky has a black eye, which she said she got when she tripped over one of the children's toys. There is a history of domestic violence.

The receptionist tells you that when Vicky left, she yelled and became angry with the children for no apparent reason.

Task: To discuss your concerns with a colleague.

YOU ARE NOT EXPECTED TO GATHER THE REST OF THE MEDICAL HISTORY DURING THIS CONSULTATION.

Points to consider:
▶ Explain succinctly your specific concerns, namely the possibility of domestic violence, and care of the children.
▶ Discuss your concerns with Vicky before alerting social services, if that is deemed to be appropriate. Always be aware of your duty of care and of the need to discuss your concerns before referring a patient to social services.
▶ Contact the health visitor and make relevant enquiries.
▶ You may suggest that they speak to Vicky about their concerns and discuss whether she requires support if she discloses violence at home.

Your notes:

Role: A GP registrar.

Setting: GP clinic.

You are talking to: Mr Jones, the father of Dylan, a 14-year-old boy.

Background information: Mr Jones has come to see you about his son's short stature. Dylan's twin sister, Rachel, is taller than him and had her first period a week ago. Mr Jones is concerned about Dylan's height, and is worried that he is being bullied at school because he is the smallest boy in his class.

Dylan is growing just above the 3rd percentile. His mid-parental height is on the 25th percentile. His recent examination showed early pubertal testes with little pubic hair. The rest of his examination was normal.

Task: To discuss constitutional growth delay with Dylan's father.

Points to consider:

‣ Explore the father's main areas of concern. He is worried about Dylan being bullied at school. He may be convinced that Dylan is shorter than his twin sister because of a disease condition that has not yet been diagnosed and which may require specialist input and treatment. He may demand 'growth' injections (which he read about recently in the local newspaper), and he may become upset and angry if Dylan is denied specialist referral and treatment.
‣ Discuss Dylan's predicted final height.
‣ Empathise with the father's concerns.
‣ As Dylan has now started puberty, reassure his father that growth and puberty will now proceed normally.
‣ Explain that Dylan's twin sister is not an identical twin, and that girls often start puberty earlier than boys.
‣ Offer advice about the timescale of likely growth.

▶ Explore the father's own pubertal growth history.
▶ Offer advice on addressing the problem of bullying.

Your notes:

This is a 9-minute station consisting of spoken interaction. You will have up to 2 minutes before the start of the station to read this sheet and prepare yourself. You may make notes on the paper provided.

When the bell sounds you will be invited into the examination room. Please take this instruction sheet with you. The examiner will not ask questions during the 9 minutes, but will warn you when you have approximately 2 minutes left.

You are not required to examine a patient.

The encounter should be focused on the task: you will be penalised for asking irrelevant questions or providing superfluous information. You will be marked on your ability to communicate, not the speed with which you convey information. You may not have time to complete the communication.

Role: Paediatric registrar.

Setting: Side-room on a busy neonatal unit.

You are talking to: Mrs Lowmass, mother of Aimee.

Background information: Aimee was born at 27 weeks' gestation via emergency Caesarean section, due to maternal pre-eclampsia. She is now 3 weeks old. She was initially ventilated for 4 days and required CPAP for a further 7 days. She is now self-ventilating in 1.0 l nasal cannula oxygen. She has had a stable course and is tolerating nasogastric feeds. The neonatal unit is full and you are expecting the delivery of 25-week twins that afternoon. The decision has been made to transfer Aimee to a smaller district general hospital 20 miles away, as she is the most stable baby in the unit, and does not require intensive care.

Task: To inform Mrs Lowmass that Aimee will be transferred later that day to another neonatal unit, and to try to address any concerns that she may have about this decision.

Points to consider:

 A likely scenario is that Mrs Lowmass will become upset and angry that you are transferring Aimee.

- ❯ Remember to offer her support in terms of having a partner or friend present, as well as a familiar member of the nursing team.
- ❯ Explain the reason why it has been decided to transfer Aimee as opposed to another baby.
- ❯ Acknowledge that this is a difficult time for the mother, as she will have formed relationships at this unit with medical and nursing staff, and possibly with other families on the unit.
- ❯ Try to present this scenario in a positive light. Aimee is stable and no longer requires an intensive-care cot. She is making excellent progress, and this is a step forward.
- ❯ Gently explain that when Aimee was born she needed the facilities and skills that this unit could offer her, and now that she is managing to breathe without any support, this same opportunity needs to be offered to another baby.
- ❯ Emphasise that Aimee will receive the same standard of care as she did before, and that it will be possible for the parents to maintain contact with the staff at this unit.
- ❯ Ask the mother whether she has any particular concerns or questions (e.g. about travelling time and/or distance, family commitments with regard to care of other siblings, financial constraints). These can all be addressed individually, and support can be offered where appropriate.
- ❯ Finally, explain the transfer arrangements to the mother, and offer to speak to her again once she has had some time to think about the situation.

Your notes:

This is a 9-minute station consisting of spoken interaction. You will have up to 2 minutes before the start of the station to read this sheet and prepare yourself. You may make notes on the paper provided.

When the bell sounds you will be invited into the examination room. Please take this instruction sheet with you. The examiner will not ask questions during the 9 minutes, but will warn you when you have approximately 2 minutes left.

You are not required to examine a patient.

The encounter should be focused on the task: you will be penalised for asking irrelevant questions or providing superfluous information. You will be marked on your ability to communicate, not the speed with which you convey information. You may not have time to complete the communication.

Role: Paediatric registrar.

Setting: Side-room in the neonatal intensive-care unit.

You are talking to: Mr and Mrs Carmichael, the parents of Ajay.

Background information: Ajay was born at 39 weeks' gestation via planned Caesarean section. He has a congenital diaphragmatic hernia. He is ventilated, but his condition has remained stable since birth. He is due to be transferred to the regional surgical centre later today, and his parents are fully aware of the planned surgical procedure. They have asked to speak to you before they leave. Mr Carmichael has read on the Internet that some babies who undergo this procedure need to be placed on extracorporeal membrane oxygenation (ECMO) post-operatively. The parents are very worried and would like to discuss this with you.

Task: To talk to Mr and Mrs Carmichael about their concerns, and to try to answer any questions they may have.

: Points to consider:

▶ This could potentially be a very difficult discussion if you have little knowledge of ECMO. However, it is reasonable to state this clearly and then to describe how you would then go on to address the parents' concerns.

▶ Before you start this discussion with the parents, you need to ask yourself the question 'What do I know about ECMO?'

▶ If you have a sound knowledge base or have previously worked at an ECMO centre, you will be comfortable answering their questions.

▶ You understand that they have read about ECMO on the Internet.

▶ You may be in a position where you need to acknowledge that this is very difficult for the parents, and that reading information on the Internet can be very frightening. If you do not have any information to give to them, be honest and say that you do not have experience of this, but that you are in a position to find out and come back to them.

▶ Offer to talk to your consultant, who will be able to explain the procedure more easily.

▶ The regional surgical team would be able to offer the parents further information and support once Ajay has been transferred. Offer to contact the receiving unit prior to transfer, so that they are able to give the parents an opportunity to talk.

▶ Explain the absolute basics of ECMO. The machine works like a heart–lung bypass machine. It takes over the work of the heart and/or lungs, and so gives the damaged organ chance to recover.

▶ Cannulae (large tubes) are inserted into the baby's large vessels, and blood is then removed and passed through the machine, where carbon dioxide is removed and oxygen is added, just as would normally be done by the lungs. The blood is then pumped back to the baby.

▶ There are risks associated with the use of ECMO, but the procedure is performed by experts in the field. If you are asked to name the specific risks, these are sepsis, blood clots and intraventricular haemorrhage.

▶ Whichever route you have taken, finally clarify whether this has resolved the parents' concerns, and ask whether there is anything else that is worrying them.

▶ Offer them further meetings and written information as appropriate.

Your notes:

This is a 9-minute station consisting of spoken interaction. You will have up to 2 minutes before the start of the station to read this sheet and prepare yourself. You may make notes on the paper provided.

When the bell sounds you will be invited into the examination room. Please take this instruction sheet with you. The examiner will not ask questions during the 9 minutes, but will warn you when you have approximately 2 minutes left.

You are not required to examine a patient.

The encounter should be focused on the task: you will be penalised for asking irrelevant questions or providing superfluous information. You will be marked on your ability to communicate, not the speed with which you convey information. You may not have time to complete the communication.

Role: Paediatric registrar working in a busy district general hospital.

Setting: Doctor's office.

You are talking to: Dr Michael Jones, an ST6 paediatric trainee.

Background information: You have worked with Michael for the last 3 months. You have a difficult professional relationship with him, as you feel that he continually criticises you in front of both patients and colleagues. He alters the management plans that you have made for patients on the ward round without discussing this with you first. You know that a number of other colleagues also find him difficult to work with; he is not a team player. More recently it has been noted that he is coming to work late. You have decided to try to talk things through with him before approaching senior staff for help.

Task: To talk to Michael, and to explain why you feel that this conversation is necessary and how things can possibly change in the future.

Points to consider:

▶ Talking to colleagues is always difficult. Be honest and try to find a way forward which will benefit the whole team and the patients.
▶ Remember that if at any point the situation becomes very

aggressive or uncomfortable, you can offer to seek impartial advice from a senior colleague who may be able to act as a mediator in this difficult situation.

▶ There is no right or wrong way to approach this discussion, but try not to adopt an aggressive attitude towards Michael, as this will immediately alienate him from you.

▶ Perhaps you could say something along the lines of 'I was wondering whether we could get a drink and try to have a chat about why things seem to be so uncomfortable between us at the moment.'

▶ Be honest, and say that you are finding it quite difficult to work alongside him at present, and that you have been upset by some of his actions at work.

▶ An open-ended question may be useful – for example, 'Are things at home or at work difficult at the moment?'

▶ Ask whether there is something in particular that you have done which may have upset him. If there is something he feels that you have done, again try not to be defensive, but listen to him and think things through before answering.

▶ If you feel that the conversation is going well, continue until you reach mutual ground. Try to agree a way forward and how you can work better together and as a team.

▶ On the other hand, if you feel that Michael is not willing or able to discuss the situation with you, say that it may be best to leave things alone for now, and perhaps suggest speaking to your educational/clinical supervisor or a trusted senior member of staff.

Your notes:

Index